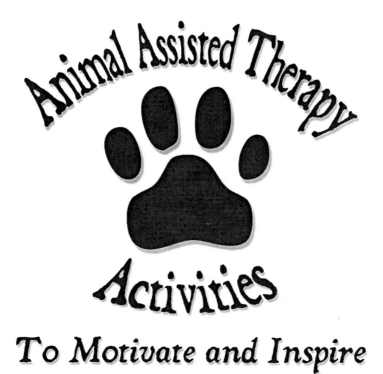

Animal Assisted Therapy Activities

To Motivate and Inspire

D1603838

Nancy Lind

Copyright Notices

Legal Notices

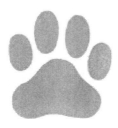

Dedication

For that original group of fifteen children who wisely showed me the many ways we could better their lives with the dogs. They were the driving force which led to the formation of the activities described in this book. These activities were designed around the skills needed to progress toward the fulfillment of the goals for which they were striving. Through their persistence to achieve, they provided the stimulus to keep me searching for new ways to challenge and motivate them.

For all the dogs who patiently showed all the skills and goals that could be accomplished through them, who persistently taught me that my job was to hold the lead, carry the suitcase, and follow their lead. Because in their wisdom they have shown that they have the instincts, patience, and skills to meet the task in front of them.

For all the teams that have carried on the tradition of working with their dogs and program participants. That only confirms what has gone before can only continue to grow to even greater heights.

It is to all of you that I respectfully dedicate this work.

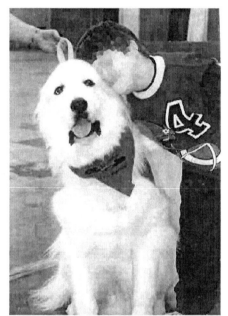

Happy dog, happy friend.

CONTENTS

Chapter		Page

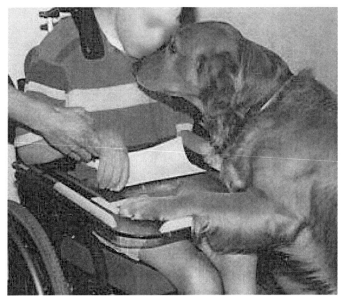

Boomer motivates a friend to stretch his arm out to pet him.

Introduction

For approximately 27 years of my professional career, I worked with special needs individuals. Originally I worked with TMH (Trainable Mentally Handicapped) persons and then, in the early 1990's, I began working with Severe and Profoundly Handicapped children.

During this time, I began to read about the use of therapy dogs in working with special needs individuals. I was then taking obedience classes with one of my dogs, Ashley. I approached a number of the people in my group and discussed the possibility of reaching out to the children in my school, as my Administrator was also interested in the program and willing to give it a shot.

We began with a "show" for the entire school in which we allowed the children to pet and interact with the dogs. I immediately noticed two things. First, the children were reaching for the leashes. They were initiating interaction with the dogs. Second, I noticed that the dogs were responding very deliberately with the children. They seemed to know that this was something important and that they had a very special task to perform with these kids.

Learning life skills through play, with dogs

From that point forward, the program began to take shape. Of our group of seven teams, (each consisting of one handler and one "therapy dog"), two teams started with two or three groups of kids, rotating on a 20 to 30 minute schedule. Building on the theory that important life skills are often learned through play, we soon learned that tasks we had been struggling to teach in the classroom became much easier with the introduction of our canine assistants.

For example, the kids immediately began to respond to the concepts of taking turns and paying attention when it meant that failure to do so resulted in their missing their turn with the dogs. After the ground rules had been established, we began to move on to more structured and task-specific games.

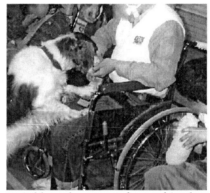

Ashley takes a treat from a friend.
(Notice children waiting for their turn)

One of the most difficult daily routines I faced in working with the severe and profoundly handicapped population was the preparation of the children to face the bitter Chicago winters at the end of the school day. Every day was a frustrating trial of shoving unresponsive fingers into gloves or mittens as the children passively, or not so passively, endured my ministrations. Then, one day, we began to play a game with the dogs in which the dog took the hats and mittens off the children. What fun! The kids were thrilled when the dogs approached them to take off their hats and gloves, but first they had to put the hats and gloves on for the dogs to steal. Suddenly a task that they had endured to have performed for them took on a new focus. Not only did they cooperate to have the items placed on their bodies, but in some cases they learned to do it themselves.

Now, not only did they become more involved in the daily task, but in some cases they learned that they actually could accomplish a task themselves! In something so very simple, the doors were now thrown open to the possibility that these kids could actually control something in their own environment.

Other Skills

These same concepts are applicable to so many different aspects of the special needs individual's daily living. Games with the dogs can be used to teach daily living skills such as dressing, the use of utensils or personal hygiene; physical strengthening through brushing, petting and walking the dogs; self-confidence through the ability to communicate with the dog through hand and voice signals to which the dog responds; and a great variety of other cognitive skills depending on the needs of the population being visited.

The "trick" to working with this population is finding the games that will address the issues of the group. To that end, I have put together this book with a number of the skills and activities that I have found to work with my students since the beginning of these programs in 1987.

I have grouped these skills in sections to help focus on a specific task. However, you will find that many of the tasks can be used to achieve a variety of goals. It is up to you to find the tools that most readily spark the interest of the children or individuals with whom you are working.

For instance, regarding Attention to Task/Tracking: When participants visually track the activity when they are attending to task, and when they continue to track the activity from participant to participant, the activity brings an added benefit of learning from watching others perform the same task over and over, thus benefitting from the multiple demonstrations. In the case of apprehension/fear of dogs, they start to gather confidence and courage from watching the successful completion of tasks from their peers.

These skills are intended to help you get started in your work with this population. You can take what you learn here and expand the activities as you become more comfortable with the goals you are trying to reach with each individual. The best tool you have is the ability to observe. Observe other teams, observe the children with whom you are working, and most of all, observe your canine teammate. Frequently you will find that your furry friend has an intuitive knowledge of just what the individual you are working with needs the most! Frequently, you will learn your best "tricks" from your four-legged partner!

Above all, have fun!

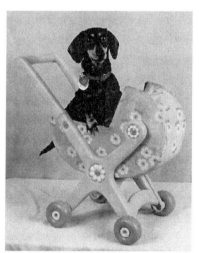

Photo by Barb Zurawski

Doozer waits for a ride in her buggy.

Benefits

The following are just some of the many benefits which result from the use of animal assisted therapy activities:

Cognitive
> Attention to Task
> Color identification
> Directional/Positional concepts
> Numerical concepts
> Reading
> Sequencing

Daily Living/Self Help
> Caring for others
> Clean up skills
> Feeding skills
> Safety

Language
> Communicating with others
> Following verbal directions
> Verbalizing wants and needs

Motor
> Balance
> Fine Motor skills
> Hand/Eye coordination
> Mobility
> Motor planning
> Range of motion
> Upper body movement/control

Social
    Control
    Cooperation/Teamwork
    Play Skills
    Self Control

All of these skills and benefits, their related animal assisted therapy activities, and where to find them, are listed in the Appendix at the end of this book.

It is my intention that you find this book a useful, informative guide, to make your therapy visits the best they can be, while enjoying every minute of the experience.

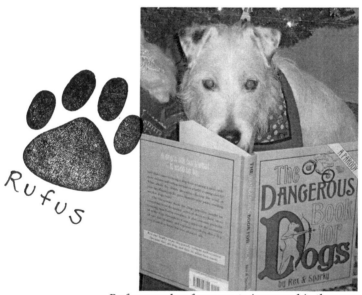

Rufus searches for ways to improve his therapy visits.

The Therapy Visit

In Animal Assisted Therapy (AAT), the volunteer and his/her animal come to work with the person in a variety of selected activities that are open-ended and non-judgmental. The objective is to find ways to allow the individual to participate. This focus and concentration on ability rather than disability, appears to be the motivating factor that allows the participant to improve and realize his/her capabilities.

Extra effort is made for the dog

For the dog, a person will make the extra effort to complete the activity, to develop skills and strengths, to build on and to increase his own self-confidence in his abilities. With the introduction of the dog to the routine, the person often forgets his limitations and is motivated to improve his/her abilities without conscious recognition of the process. These skills learned in play with the dog allow the participant to overcome his limitations and lack of motivation and improves his ability to succeed to higher goals without focusing on the disabilities that prevented him from participating in traditional recreation and leisure activities.

No one likes to be told what their shortcomings are and have them demonstrated time and time again to reinforce those deficits to others. Instead, isn't it much more constructive to focus on the capabilities we do have and to nurture those talents in the development of new skills? I am convinced that the reason we sometimes see dramatic results is that the human and animal team interact as a whole and directly *with* the individual on a give-and-take basis, allowing ALL participants to be part of the session and its outcome.

Forget about limitations and expectations

It is my thought that the success of AAT is derived from this unique interaction on a thoroughly even playing field devoid of opinion, expectation or pre-conceived notions concerning the abilities/disabilities of the participant. This freedom from expectations and limitations allows us to look below the surface and let new skills, thoughts and abilities emerge. It allows the entire interaction to develop into an event that is part of the person's life and not an activity which may get lost in the act of performing for someone else.

AAT is *an invitation to look deeply, to ponder, and then let the doing come out of the activity.* Participants can forget about limitations and expectations and enter into a challenge of achievement for self, practice without dwelling on the outcome, and focus on the experience itself. Being mindful is not about doing it perfectly, but about doing it the best one can at that moment, even if it isn't "perfect" by others' standards. AAT is about being able to acknowledge accomplishment and to come away from that experience with something that helps the individual to try in a different, perhaps better, way.

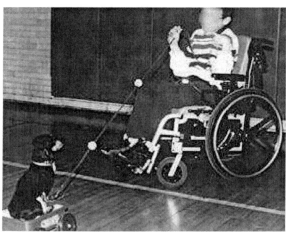

Taking Doozer for a ride.

3

Is Your Dog a Therapy Dog?

Needed: A well-mannered pet who is friendly and comfortable in all types of surroundings (or at least those in which you intend to work).

Pre-requisite skill: Willingness to learn.

Walking: The dog should be able to walk mannerly at one's side on a loose lead. He should demonstrate willingness, attention and cooperation to its owner's movements, turns, stops and starts, etc.

Remaining in place: While visiting, this could be either a sit, down or stand, whichever works best during the visit. It is to the handler's advantage to have his dog able to perform all three positions on command.

Settle down: The dog should demonstrate the ability to calm down and remain under control while visiting a facility.

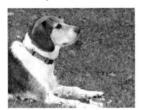

Attention: The dog should be attentive to the handler/participants' commands.

Photo by Linda Grundeman
Pretzel pays attention.

Grooming: Dogs should always be clean, well-groomed, free of any discharges (eye, nose or in season), free of any odors (good or bad), sprays or powders of any kind, and free of any parasites (fleas, ticks, etc.). Remember, a number of the children you will be working with have wide reaching physical and/or behavioral challenges. The child may have allergies or may be hypersensitive to scent as a result of certain types of treatment (such as chemotherapy).

Disposition: Willingness to interact with strangers, enjoy being petted, fondled and receiving attention from others.

As a note to competitors in various fields of dog activities (such as conformation, obedience, agility, and fly ball), animal-assisted visits are not to be viewed as training grounds for your other activities. You may find, however, that the performance of these activities might be entertaining to those you visit.

It is important to remember that those you are visiting would not like to see strict training and correction taking place. Some of the individuals you may work with have been the subject of abuse, either verbal or physical, or both. It can often be very distressing to the participant to witness a correction, especially when he has no frame of reference in which to understand that the correction is not overly harsh. If you are seeking a level of perfection and precision at all times when you are competing, you might want to refrain from using these activities in a therapy session where you cannot make corrections. You might also use different commands for the same behavior to help your dog know when they are free to perform and when they are working with precision.

It's O.K. to make a mistake

Also, remember that perfection is not necessary in this setting. In fact, when the dog makes a mistake, it is a useful demonstration to the participants that perfection is neither expected nor required for the dog to do a good job. It's okay for the dog to need a little help to achieve the desired goal, and sometimes, as with people, we just have to find another way to communicate what we are looking for. Not every dog will perform the same activity in exactly the same way, just as no two people will do every task in exactly the same way.

Preparation

For dogs to do a wide variety of animal-assisted activities and therapies and to be of maximum benefit to the participant with whom they are interacting, they need to feel comfortable so that they can work relaxed.

AAT dogs should be exposed as much as possible to many different indoor/outdoor places that have a wide variety of floor surfaces, noises and activities. Exposure to a variety of entrances, stairways, elevators, etc. should be handled before starting actual therapy visits. You will find that some dogs can be overly stressed by any number of things and will perform in a limited fashion or not at all when they have been exposed to an uncomfortable situation.

Your dog should be fully at ease and relaxed when performing AAT visits in a clinical or recreational setting to be of maximum benefit to the people you are visiting. You will notice that, at the end of the sessions, they are usually quite tired and will most likely sleep soundly in the car on the way home. During the session, it is your responsibility to monitor your animal's emotional and physical status for stress, thirst, temperature, tiredness, etc.

Stress

If you see signs of stress (excessive yawning, lack of attention, sweaty paws, shedding, etc.) or if your canine partner is not performing well on a particular day, you should consider taking a break or sitting off to the side for the remainder of the session. These animals don't punch a time clock, and it is important for the handler to know when it is time to move on or quit.

For the dogs to be able to participate on a regular schedule, they too have to enjoy their part in the whole animal-assisted therapy event. Lack of eagerness upon entering a program might indicate that your canine partner is overworked, ill, or just needs to take a "vacation" from his "work".

You're a team

You have a desire to visit with your pet and you have a well-mannered pet that enjoys visiting people. It might be desirable to brush up on your pet's obedience skills. If you want to do therapeutic programs, you will need to add more skills to your repertoire.

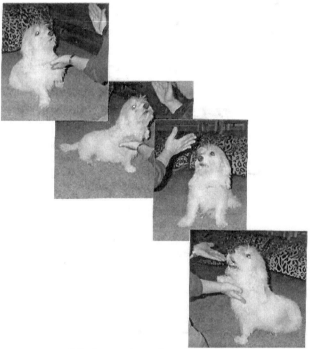

PG plays pat-a-cake with a friend.

Where to Find Training

To find local testing organizations/testers, contact the following national registries. Local dog obedience training organizations and animal welfare groups might be helpful in referring you to the groups actively doing therapy dog visits in your area.

Take and pass one of the national therapy tests. Complete and send in the required paperwork and fees.

Delta Society – Pet Partners
875 124th Avenue, N.E, Suite #101
Bellevue, WA 98005-2531
425-679-5500
425-679-5539 (fax)
Email: petpartners@deltasociety.org
Website: www.deltasociety.org

Therapy Dogs International, Inc.
88 Bartley Road
Flanders, NJ 07836
973 252-9800
973 252-7171 (fax)
Email: tdi@gti.net
Website: www.tdi-dog.org

Therapy Dogs, INC.
P.O. Box 20227
Cheyenne, WY 82003
877 843-7364
307-432-0272
307 638-2079 (fax)
Email: therapydogsinc@qwestoffice.net
Website: www.therapydogs.com

The following websites may assist you in finding other local Animal assisted Therapy Groups in your area:

www.dogplay.com

www.landofpuregold.com

www.therapypets.com/index.html

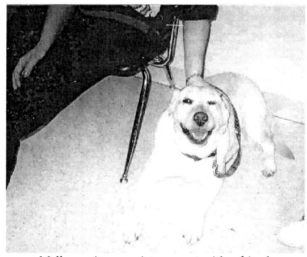

Mellow enjoys a quiet moment with a friend.

Your Dog is a Therapy Dog

After passing the test there are many types of programs in which you and your dog may participate. Among them are:

Day care (children/adult)
Detention facilities
Hospice/home visits
Hospitals – therapeutic/rehab (group/individual)
Nursing homes
Park/recreational facilities/day camps
Psychiatric facilities
Residential facilities/room visits
Libraries
Schools and vocational training programs (pre-school, high school, regular/special education)

AAT is designed to work under the direction of the facility staff to address motor, language, behavioral, social, self help, visual, and cognitive skills and to increase memory, attention span, responsibility, confidence and safety.

Consider the following points in selecting places to visit:
- Therapeutic or visiting sessions
- Quiet or highly active
- Single dog or group visits
- Special education or regular education
- Children or adult
- Pre-school, grade school or high school age

It is important to note that you and your animal must feel comfortable that you have the skills required to meet the facility's and participants' needs.

Decide whether you want to work independently or as part of an existing local therapy dog group.

If visiting independently:
- Determine the types of groups and facilities for which you and your pet are best suited.
- Locate the facilities that might want your visits.
- Learn facilities' needs, rules and protocol.
- Identify/train the skills that you will need.
- Find a local therapy dog training class. (Check local library or internet.)
- Expose your pet to high traffic areas, parks, schools, train stations, shopping areas.
- Read and learn the rules of your national registry.

Or **join an existing therapy group** in your area, with programs already in place.

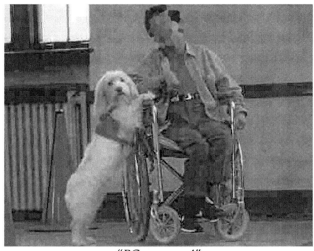

"PG, paws up!"

Visiting (Disability) Etiquette

- Remember that you are their guest.
- Your animal is the key to the visit. You are to facilitate the visit or skill interaction.
- The participants have the right to refuse or accept the visit.
- The team must respect the participant's personal space (his/her lap, chair, bed, walker). Do not lean, sit or hang on them or their equipment.
- Provide covers (sheets, rubber shelf liners) for laps, beds, etc. for protection and cleanliness.
- Treat participants in a considerate manner. Do not patronize, belittle, or show overt signs of affection.
- When offering assistance, guide, rather than propel or lead.
- Ask if they want help before giving assistance. Once accepted, follow their instructions.
- Interact directly with the person, rather than through a third person.
- Get the person's attention. Look and speak directly to the participant.
- Give each participant your unhurried attention without ignoring the rest of the group.
- Keep your manner encouraging, rather than correcting.
- Keep the action moving at a steady pace.
- Be considerate of the extra time needed for their responses or any barriers that present themselves.

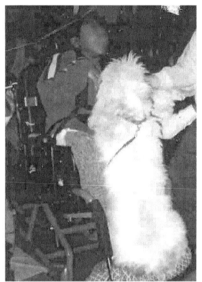

PG sits on footrest while visiting a friend.

Be Prepared for Each Visit

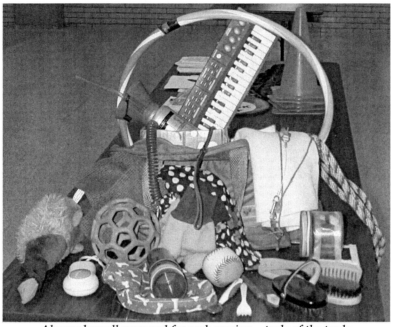

Always be well prepared for each session – tools of the trade.

Possible Items for Bag of Tricks

Cones, rope, cups, hoop, bowling game, different sized balls, treats, fork and/or spoon, toothbrush, grooming brush, comb, curlers and hairclips, spray bottle, dress up costume, musical instruments, cleanup supplies, water and bowl, extra leashes, books (read to the dogs), massage, blindfold, treat jar for tricks, and much, much more. Use your imagination and watch your teammates for new ideas. A good source for equipment is the children's toy aisle in any department store, garage sales and secondhand stores. Be sure to keep safety precautions and cleanliness of all equipment in mind as you prepare for the needs of the participants of each program.

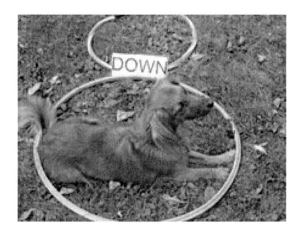

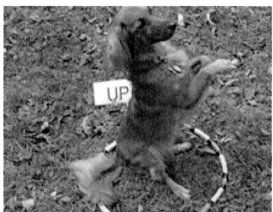

Photos by Linda Grundeman
The life of a therapy dog has its "ups and downs."

Getting Started-Basic AAT Concepts & Activities

- Have Fun!

- Be Adaptable!

- Be Safe!

- Be Creative!

- Be Challenging!

- Be Entertaining!

- Be a Distraction!

- Be a Diversion!

- Be Enjoyable!

- Mistakes are O.K.

- Non-obedience Training is O.K.

- Games are meant to be FUN!

"No Trick" dog tricks

Throughout this book, you will find activities and tricks which I classify as "no trick" dog tricks. Many of these tricks are the old standbys used to entertain family and friends. Dogs want to be occupied and, for the owner's peace of mind, it may as well be constructive. If not, the dog will be left to his own devices to occupy his time which usually does not meet with the owner's idea of constructive activity.

Tricks can be a useful way of earning praise, the owner's attention, and possibly feeling useful. Dogs have been bred to work. If you don't own a flock of sheep, fields to hunt, varmints to chase or estates to guard, you need to develop your own constructive work schedule for your canine companion. After your four-pawed friend finishes his lessons in basic manners, don't let him become a sleeping dog. Use tricks to make him your helper, entertainer and otherwise great companion.

"No trick" tricks are basically tricks which your dog usually does on his own. All that is needed is for you to add a command to the behavior and praise it. Watch your dog and note the behavior (stretch, scratch his back on the floor, sneeze, scratch, yawn, shake, etc.)

For example, when your dog shakes a toy, you say "good shake" and give praise. Repeat this each time your dog does it and soon you can tell your dog to shake when you give him his toy, and he will respond on command. *Voila!* Your best friend has a new trick in his portfolio. And the tricks get easier to teach as the habit becomes ingrained. Each time he learns a new trick, learning the next trick becomes that much easier.

Here are some "no trick" tricks:

Bow	Catch	Wearing a costume
Turn around	Ride a wagon	Ride battery toy
Reading	Sing/talk	Spelling
Foreign language	Sneeze	Answer question
Eat off spoon/fork	Kiss	Wag tail
Paw tricks		

Have lots of activities "in your bag"

When providing therapeutic activities, it is necessary that you and your dog have a lot of different activities in your bag. It is important for teams to recognize that it takes more than four paws, a wet nose, and a wagging tail to effect a change in the people you are visiting. A team has to come up with a variety of activities when the facility requests that motor, behavioral, social, self-help, language, cognitive and/or visual skills be addressed. When planning activities, one should also try to incorporate safety, memory, attention skills, and activities that will build feelings of responsibility and confidence.

All dogs can learn a repertoire of activities. Some do it easier than others. Be very creative in the activities you choose to use. The important thing to remember is the number of activities your dog will do for those they are visiting, not that your dog has to do the very same activity that the other teams around you are doing.

It's a process

Teaching your dog activities is a building process. The dog has to learn the teaching process. Once they learn there is a command/signal, their response, followed by your praise/treat, will become easier for them. If your dog likes to fetch, see how many variations of fetching you can develop. If your dog is very good at finding treats, see how many activities you can come up with (such as the cup game and bowling). Hide treats or a toy in the children's socks, pockets or sleeves for the dogs to nuzzle out. If they display a natural willingness to use their paw, you can teach paw, high 5, right and left, tambourine/piano, pat-a-cake and the wave.

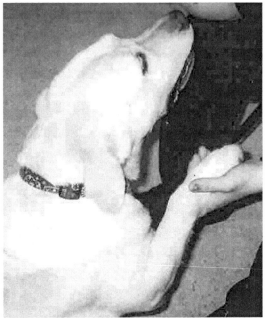

Mellow attentively gives "Paw."

One trick at a time

Just teach one trick and after your dog knows that, go on to the second trick. Occasionally, go back and reinforce the older tricks in their bag. Also plan to teach very different activities to avoid confusion with your dog (such as trying to teach him how to speak and sneeze).

Give Kiss

Skills needed:	Lick on command.
Equipment:	None.
Directions:	Handler touches participant's hand and directs dog to it.
Teaching tips:	Place small amount of cheese on the back of the participant's hand and point to it while giving the dog the "kiss" command.
Benefits:	Communicating with others, Verbalizing wants and needs, Self control.
Note:	Its best not to have the dog kiss around the face.

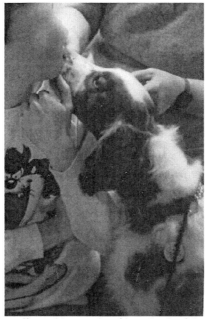

Ashley offers a kiss on the side or back of the neck.

Nothing Trick

Skills needed:	Down-stay on side or back.
Equipment:	Optional.
Directions:	Voice/signal to down.
Variations:	1) Command to sleep or take a nap and optionally cover with a blanket.
	2) "Tummy rub" if positioned on back.
Benefits:	Directional/positional, Sequencing, Verbalizing wants and needs, Upper Body movement/control, Control.
Note:	The command "play dead" is not recommended for most of the populations you might visit.

Costumes and Dress-up

Silly stunts and costumes certainly have a place in your therapy dog's list of tricks and talents. They serve as a real ice breaker and make people laugh and feel happy and relaxed. In some cases, a silly costume can make larger dogs a little less intimidating to those who are not accustomed to being around large animals. Finally, they help you keep the line of communication open between you and your dog and can be a signal to your dog that he is "going to work".

Costumes can consist of wearing a simple hat, scarf or tie, or they can become more elaborate to include tee shirts, sweatshirts with funny pictures and sayings or holiday costumes. Use your imagination and make an activity out of allowing the participants to dress the dog and themselves up for part of the visit. Holidays and theme days can also serve as inspiration for costume ideas. Some of your tricks can be an additional source for ideas to develop costumes to dress up your stunts, such as a fancy fur stole and pearls for the female canines in your group, a tuxedo for the piano playing pooch, or local sports team shirts and hats for the four-legged basketball players.

Use sports, holidays, food, animals, or any inspiration to fire your creativity. Children's and infant departments of resale or second-time-around stores are good places to look for costume ideas and props.

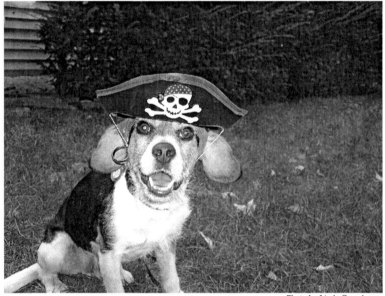

Photo by Linda Grundeman

Pretzel the Pirate.

Play Piano

Skills needed:	Paw or touch command.
Equipment:	Toy piano or keyboard.
Directions:	Participant gives dog sit or down command to position him by piano and then gives command to play the piano.
Variations:	1) Command for fast, slow or stop. 2) Command for 1 or 2 paws. 3) Combined efforts of more dogs with instruments.
Benefits:	Attention to Task, Directional/positional, Sequencing, Following verbal directions, Verbalizing wants & needs, Motor planning, Upper body movement/control, Control, Play skills.

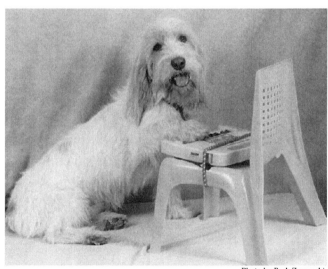

Photo by Barb Zurawski

PG plays piano.

Play Tambourine

Skills needed:	Paw or touch command.
Equipment:	Tambourine.
Directions:	Participant gives dog sit or down command to position him. Participant holds tambourine by strap in front of dog and then gives command to "play the tambourine".
Variations:	Command for fast, slow or stop.
Benefits:	Attention to task, Directional/positional, Numerical concepts, Sequencing, Communicating with others, Following verbal directions, Verbalizing wants and needs, Fine motor skills, Hand/eye coordination, Motor planning, Upper body movement/control, Control, Cooperation/teamwork, Play skills.

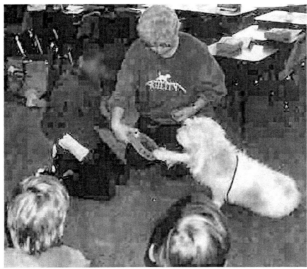

PG plays tambourine with her friends.

Motorcycle Rider

Skills needed:	Sit/stay on moving object.
Equipment:	Battery-operated motorcycle, wagon, wheelchair or other moving vehicle.
Directions:	Trainer positions dog on apparatus. Participant gives dog command to "stay" and then operates apparatus (by turning on motorcycle, pulling wagon or pushing wheelchair).
Variations:	Participant can dress dog in appropriate costume (goggles).
Benefits:	Directional/positional, Caring for others, Verbalizing wants and needs, Balance, Mobility, Motor planning, Upper body movement/control, Control, Play skills.

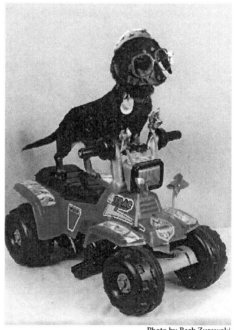

Photo by Barb Zurawski

Doozer rides the motorcycle.

30

Read

Skills needed:	None
Equipment:	Poster/cue card with very large print on both sides ("wag tail" on front, "sit" on back). Handler should orient lettering for convenient "flipping" of the sign.
Directions:	1) Front of sign is held at dog's eye level with a motion/signal prompting the dog to stand and wag tail.
	2) Sign is flipped over with a motion/signal prompting the dog to sit.
	3) Repeat steps 1 and 2.
Benefits:	Attention to task, Reading, Sequencing, Communicating with others, Fine motor skills, Upper body movement/control, Confidence, Control, Cooperation/teamwork.

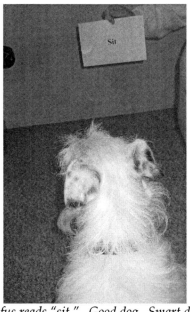

Rufus reads "sit." Good dog. Smart dog.

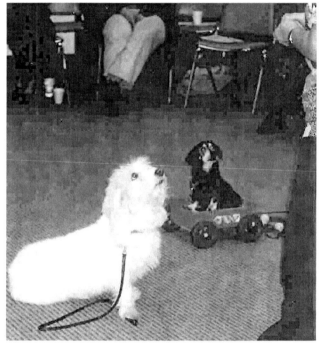

PG & Doozer watch for next hand signal.

Hand Signals

Using hand signals with skills and tricks:

- Gives those who are non-verbal a means to interact.
- Shows excellent cause and effect encouraging the use of sign language as a means of everyday communication.
- Motivates and encourages use of specific parts of the body to aid in co-ordination and physical movement.
- Encourages vocalization when hand and voice commands are used in conjunction with each other.
- Allows for sequencing and chaining commands together to teach more advanced use of language.
- Gives the handler non-verbal control of their dog and allows prompting their dog when needed.
- Encourages your dog to maintain eye contact with you.

Hand signals add an additional mode of communication and also provide the motivation to:
- Use the upper body to give the signal.
- Provide a good bridge in learning human sign language.

It is important that you do not rush your intervention. Allow the participant the time and opportunity to work out problems, try different techniques, and become more assertive.

A hand signal should be paired with the voice command

As your dog learns each skill or trick, a hand signal should be paired with the voice command. The choice of the signal is up to each trainer. The trainer must remember to keep the hand signals consistent so the dog is able to understand them. When planning the signals to use for a variety of movements and actions, think of the various single and paired actions with arms, hands, and fingers. Think of motions which involve reaching, extension, rotation, circling, swinging, bending, oppositional motion, mirroring, and so on. Movements and actions can be used in a therapeutic setting to encourage movement on the part of the participant you and your animal are visiting.

<u>Skill:</u>	<u>Signal:</u>
Sit	Right hand facing palm forward at side, raised at the elbow to touch the right shoulder.
Down	Forefinger touching the floor or hand over head, palm facing forward. Hand is lowered to the side with a straight arm.

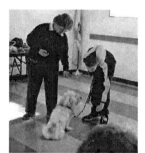

Participant signals PG "Down."

Come	Right hand is held straight out to the side with palm facing forward. Arm is swept across the body to touch the left shoulder or clap hands or pat your thigh with one hand.

Roll over   After placing the dog in a down, make a small circular motion with finger/hand in front of dog's nose (clockwise for rollover to right and counter clockwise for roll to left.

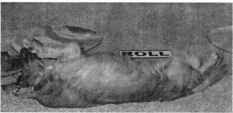

Photo By Linda Grundeman
Beaner demonstrates "Roll Over."

Sit up   Holding treat in fingers, hand is extended to the dog's nose and then it is moved back over the dog's head until the dog is in sit up position.

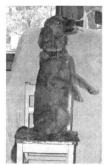

Photo by Linda Grundeman
Beaner "in balance."

Turn around   Holding treat between finger and thumb, draw a slow circle parallel to the floor leading the dog around in a circle (clockwise for circle right, counter-clockwise for circle left).

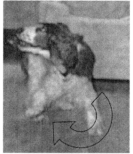

Photo by Linda Grundeman
A turn-around by Keyfer.

Speak   Open and close thumb and fingers several times
                (like the mouth of a puppet).
                Variation: Open and close index finger and
                thumb for "speak softly" and to get a quieter
                bark.

Heel   With palm facing forward, swing left hand or
                pat left leg.

Stay   Swing left hand to left side in front of dog's nose
                while coming to a stop or place palm in front of
                dog's nose while stopping.

Stand   Turn to the dog and place palm of right hand in
                front of dog's nose and move it away from the
                dog.

Give paw   Extend hand to dog as if to shake with palm up.

High five   Hand is extended in front of the dog with
                fingers pointing up and palm facing out.

Give ten   Both hands extended to dog as in High Five.

Wave   One hand stretched out in front, palm facing
                down. Move hand right and left from the wrist.

10

AAT Activities That Motivate

Ladder Walk

Skills needed:	Heel.
Equipment:	Ladder or hula hoops.
Directions:	Participant will heel dog through a ladder than is lying flat on the floor while giving "walk it" command.
Variations:	Use hula hoop or three-step practice stairs in same manner as the ladder. Participant can follow dog as deemed beneficial. When using equipment, handler should be conscious of safety precautions to prevent stumbling or falls. Staff should be present and actively monitoring participant safety.
Benefits:	Attention to task, Directional/positional, Verbalizing wants and needs, Balance, Mobility, Motor planning, Upper body movement/control, Confidence, Control, Cooperation/teamwork.

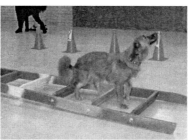

Photo by Linda Grundeman
Beaner watches handler for direction while walking the ladder.

Hoop

Skills needed:	Jump on command.
Equipment:	Hula hoop (the beads may be removed if they make the dog nervous).
Directions:	Participant holds hoop in vertical position and gives verbal/hand signal for dog to go through hoop.
Variations:	1) Team work (two participants hold hoop while third gives command). 2) Positioning of hoop (right side, left side, front, and back).
Benefits:	Attention to task, Directional/positional, Verbalizing wants and needs, Communicating with others, Motor planning, Range of motion, Upper body movement/control, Control, Positional concepts, Hand/arm strength and control

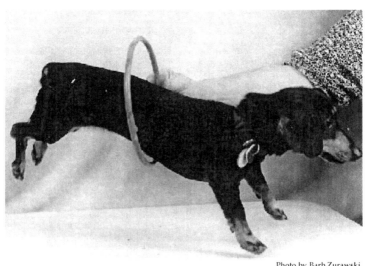

Photo by Barb Zurawski

Doozer jumps through the hoop.

Dog Pulling Wagon

Skills needed:	Fetch and pull.
Equipment:	Toy wagon with ball on pull rope.
Directions:	1) Participant gives signal and/or verbal command for dog to fetch toy on pull rope.
	2) Participant gives signal and/or verbal command for dog to "pull."
	3) Participant walks beside dog pulling wagon.
Variations:	Participant pulls dog in wagon.
Benefits:	Attention to task, Directional/positional, Communicating with others, Verbalizing wants and needs, Balance, Mobility, Motor planning, Upper body movement/control, Control, Cooperation/teamwork, Play skills.

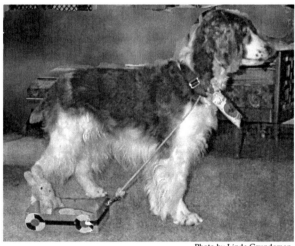

Photo by Linda Grundeman

Note: Popular trick for entertainment at demonstrations or shows. Dog should be comfortable with skills prior to introduction in session.

Weave (Izzy Dizzy)

Skills needed:	Attention to handler.
Equipment:	None.
Directions:	Participant stands with feet spread apart and uses treat to guide dog in and around his legs weaving in and out.
Variations:	1) Have dog weave around cones or weave poles.
	2) Have dog weave in and out of participants arranged in line on the floor. This could also be used as a relay if the participant passes off the leash when he reaches the end of the line. There can be two or more lines running simultaneously. You need to work out the relay logistics, perhaps using the handler to return the dog to the next participant in line.
Benefits:	Attention to task, Directional/positional, Safety, Communicating with others, Verbalizing wants and needs, Balance, Mobility, Motor planning, Range of motion, Upper body movement/control, Control, Cooperation/teamwork, Play skills, Self control.

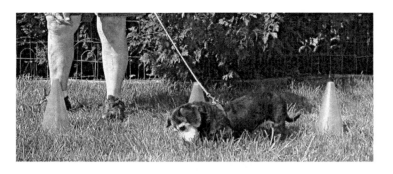

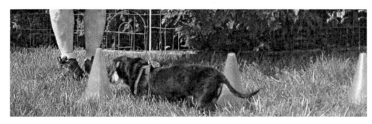

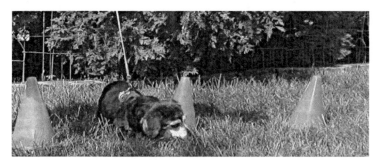

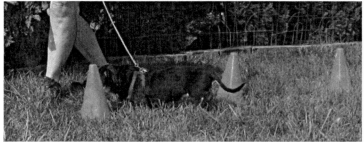

Photos By: Linda Grundeman

Doozer follows directions to weave through cones.

Catch

Skills needed:	Sit/stay and catching.
Equipment:	Object to be tossed (treat or toy).
Directions:	1) Participant gives signal and/or verbal command for dog to sit and stay.
	2) Participant walks 6-10 feet in front of dog and turns to face dog.
	3) Participant tosses object to dog with command to catch.
Variations:	Have participant move further away from dog.
Benefits:	Attention to task, Directional/positional, Sequencing, Communicating with others, Verbalizing wants and needs, Mobility, Motor planning, Range of motion, Upper body movement/control, Control, Cooperation/teamwork
Cautions:	Be sure that you are working in a clear and controlled area when performing this exercise. It is important to prevent the treat/toy from interfering with another team's activities and to prevent any possible altercations between dogs.

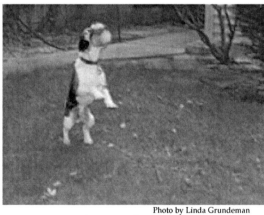

Photo by Linda Grundeman
Great catch, Pretzel!

Snake Walk

Skills needed: Attention to handler, go through, under.
Equipment: Cones, if desired.
Directions: With dog on left side, participant takes one step with right foot and commands the dog to "under" and "turn." Participant then steps with left foot and repeats commands, alternating steps.
Variations: Participant can "snake" through cones
Benefits: Attention to task, Directional/positional, Sequencing, Safety, Communicating with others, Following verbal directions, Verbalizing wants and needs, Balance, Mobility, Motor planning, Control.

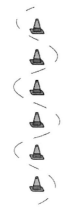

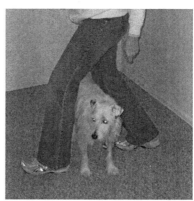

Rufus starts the "snake walk."

Carry the Basket

Skills needed:	Fetch, hold, go to.
Equipment:	Basket to carry with wrapped treats for participants.
Directions:	Trainer gives dog basket with treats and gives "go to" command. Dog goes to each participant and sits for participant to take treat from basket (especially good at holidays).
Variations:	Participants can put items in basket for dog to collect.
Benefits:	Attention to task, Directional/positional, Communicating with others, Fine motor skills, Hand/eye coordination, Cooperation/teamwork, Self control.

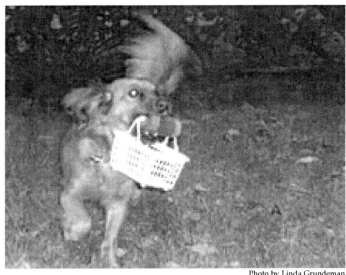

Photo by Linda Grundeman

Beaner and the Basket.

Over/Under

Skills needed:	"Crawl" and/or "jump" on command.
Equipment:	None.
Directions:	Participant gets on hands and knees. Handler gives dog "under" or "crawl" command and dog goes under participant. Participant turns and lies on his back. Handler gives dog "over" command to jump over participant.
Variations:	1) Additional participants line up to form tunnel.
	2) Another participant gives commands instead of handler.
	3) Participants line up alternating "over" and "under."
Benefits:	Attention to task, Directional/positional, Sequencing, Communicating with others, Following verbal directions, Balance, Mobility, Motor planning, Range of motion, Cooperation/teamwork, Self control.

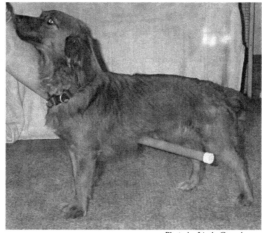

Photo by Linda Grundeman

Beaner goes "over" the baton.

45

Jump Rope

Skills needed:	"Crawl" and "jump" on command.
Equipment:	Thick, bright rope.
Directions:	Two participants hold ends of rope and third participant gives the dog the command to "jump" or "over."
Variations:	1) Two people (handler and participant) hold rope and participant gives command. 2) Command to have dog "over" and "circle" to come back.
Benefits:	Attention to task, Directional/positional, Sequencing, Communicating with others, Following verbal commands, Upper body movement/control, Control, Cooperation/teamwork.

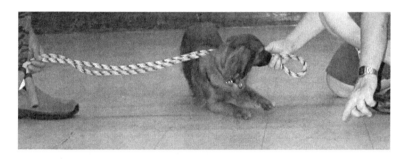

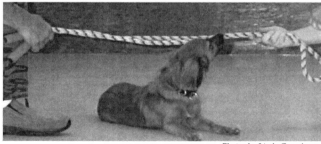

Photos by Linda Grundeman

Beaner crawls "under" the rope.

Crawl

Skills needed:	"Down" and "crawl."
Equipment:	None or chairs, tunnel, etc.
Directions:	Participant gives command for down and then crawl.
Variations:	1) Dog crawls under rope, chair or participant who is on hands and knees.
	2) Additional participants line up to form tunnel.
	3) Dogs compete with other teams to play "limbo."
Benefits:	Attention to task, Directional/positional, Sequencing, Communicating with others, Following verbal directions, Verbalizing wants and needs, Balance, Mobility, Control, Cooperation/teamwork.

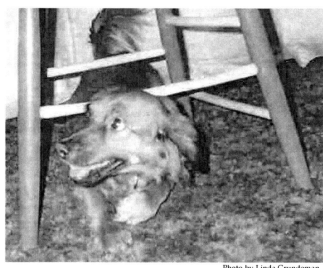

Photo by Linda Grundeman

Beaner crawls "under" the chair.

Slide

Skills needed:	"Climb" and "slide."
Equipment:	Small pre-school slide.
Directions:	Participant heels dog to ramp and gives the voice/hand signal to climb up. Participant gives command to "wait" at top and then to "slide".
Benefits:	Attention to task, Directional/positional, Sequencing, Communicating with others, Verbalizing wants and needs, Mobility, Motor planning, Upper body movement/control, Control, Cooperation/teamwork.

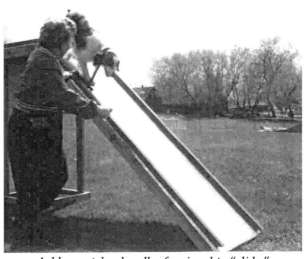

Ashley watches handler for signal to "slide."

Dance

Skills needed:	Stand on hind legs.
Equipment:	None.
Directions:	Participant gives dog voice or hand command to stand on hind legs and then uses treat to lead dog to "dance."
Variations:	Commands for "back", "forward," "right", "left". Music could be added for demos and to entertain groups of participants.
Benefits:	Verbalizing wants and needs, Balance, Hand/eye coordination, Range of motion, Upper body movement/control, Control.

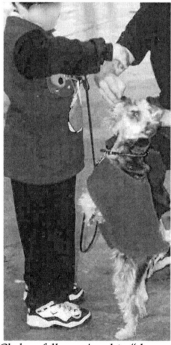

Chelsea follows signal to "dance."

Dice

Skills needed:	Tricks that are listed on the "card."
Equipment:	Large size dice, (i.e., made of foam, plush, etc). Card with list of tricks the dog can perform, numbered 2-12.
Directions:	Participant "throws" dice, then counts the dots on the dice. Participant reads the trick next to the number on the card. Participant instructs dog to perform the trick.
Benefits:	Numerical concepts, Reading, Sequencing, Communicating with others, Verbalizing wants/needs, Upper body movement/control, Control, Cooperation/teamwork, Play skills.

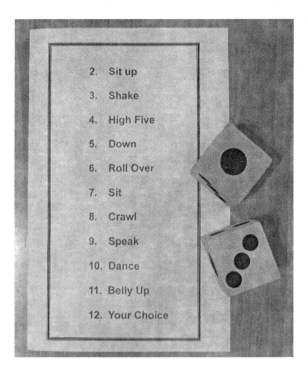

2. Sit up

3. Shake

4. High Five

5. Down

6. Roll Over

7. Sit

8. Crawl

9. Speak

10. Dance

11. Belly Up

12. Your Choice

AAT Games That Motivate

Over the years, the educational system has found that one of the most efficient and lasting ways to teach basic academic skills is through the use of games. Thus, games have moved from the gym and playground into the classroom. Games stimulate interest and purpose in learning any skill and provide the momentum to facilitate learning and allow for instruction without suffering a loss in spontaneity or creativity.

Skills, Rules and Sequencing

Games require not only the skill to be learned but also rules and sequencing of steps. In many cases, these two requirements are the very tasks the special needs community often struggles with, and these difficulties, when not addressed, cause them to be disinterested in games. They therefore fail to reap the benefits that could otherwise be recognized.

Through the participation in structured game playing, the individual will often happen upon a new skill or movement without being aware of it. In AAT, because the focus has been shifted to participation with the animal and the emphasis has been removed from the accomplishment of the task itself, the door is opened to the enjoyment of the movements or activities that the participant might have struggled with previously.

Playing games with a therapy dog helps the individual overcome the difficulty in mastering the complexity of playing a game without the social stigma of making mistakes or failing to understand the rules. In time the game allows participants to develop the necessary skills to complete the task at hand in time.

Additionally, because the participants are teamed with a canine counterpart, they learn compassion in helping another living creature to complete a task successfully. This overshadows the importance of their own personal achievement and can lessen the impact of not coming in "first".

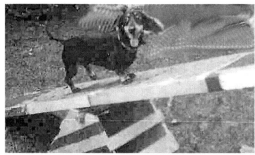

Doozer walks the "see-saw."
Agility activities are also beneficial in
game playing/skill building

It's not just a game

Games can be developed to motivate individuals to perform skills that they have long given up trying to accomplish. Often these daily skills are done by others because it takes too long for the individual to achieve the skill themselves. Additionally, games teach sharing and caring, following the rules, and cooperation. They foster sportsmanship and social values. They contribute to the participant's motor, social and emotional growth, and provide an opportunity to experiment with movement, engage in handling different types of equipment and experience activities not normally present in their school or recreation program. Most importantly, the individual should be given a forum to try, experiment, fail and succeed without judgment.

Utilization of Games Designed to Meet Specific Learning Objectives

The basic design of commonly known games is retained, but the concepts to be learned, the vocabulary used, and the playing procedures are changed to suit and address the needs of the participants and to accommodate the interaction of their canine friends.

These pages are intended to give you some ideas that may be helpful in your sessions. They are to serve as a stepping-off point for your programs and imagination.

Criteria for Choosing Games

Selecting appropriate games promotes a level of thinking needed for specific objectives. Select durable materials free of sharp edges. Consider appearance, bright colors, novel objects, portability and ease of cleaning. The content of the games should reflect the ability of a participant to compete on some level of success. The game should include **purpose, instructions/rules,** and the **necessary equipment**.

Games of all age levels can be played without belittling the participant that it is too "babyish" for them. Even developmentally delayed children view themselves as participating in activities that are appropriate to their chronological age and usually are not interested in games below their age level. Sometimes, however, with the participation of the dogs, this barrier is overlooked, possibly because the children feel in control of the activity and feel that they are assisting the dog to play the game that is within the dog's level of ability.

Prizes

This population generally does not participate in competition. In fact, due to their disabilities, they usually are deprived of the opportunity. Many love the chance to compete like and with their peers.

The prizes themselves can be as simple as different colored candy canes (color denoting degree of accomplishment), stickers, cardboard "bonus" bones, etc. In this way, the prizes can be of equal value with the color of the prize being the reward for those who strive for extra accomplishment. Games without winners and losers can be used effectively, but that should not limit the selection of games used as these children relish the opportunity to be competitive.

Also, remember that effort should be rewarded. For some of these individuals, the very act of participating in a game is an accomplishment in itself and should be recognized and encouraged.

Music

Music sets the mood and pace for many activities and should be considered as an addition to the game playing selection.

Organization

The decision regarding who gets to go first can be decided in many ways: roll of the dice, count off, rotating players, etc. With some populations, however, it must be remembered that taking turns and cooperation are some of the most important skills that the participants need to work on. Lining up, waiting in turn and volunteering are all aspects of behavior that should be incorporated in the game.

- Lines can be created with mats, colored tape, chalk, or traffic cones.
- Select games that allow for rule variations to suit the needs of your participants and their canine friends.
- Select games with rotating leaders and games that facilitate multiple winners.

Games should be modified to allow fluid play and encourage the players to work on the skills they need to improve. For example, throwing, paying attention, language skills and self-control are all developmental aspects that can be incorporated into the game playing activities.

Modification should also allow for success in the game. Remember, games are played, for the most part, to be won and lost. Rules should be set and followed. If the participants are allowed to overtly disregard the playing rules, they will be getting the wrong message and deprived of the challenge of competition.

Safety

Energetic games are not intended for timid, small, fearful or excitable participants or dogs. Care should be exercised in choosing the appropriate activity levels based upon the size and needs of the group and the space available for safe play.

The play area should be free of hazards, contained, and escape proof.

Games should stimulate cooperation. Use games at the participant's skill level. For fun, keep the games goal-oriented and, most of all, safe for the participants and the dogs. Safety first! Use mats to avoid slipping and avoid games requiring speed. Keep dogs on lead at all times, and play games that limit contact between other participants and dogs. Teams should be observant to activities going on around them, and handlers should be vigilant to prevent their dogs from interfering in another team's activity, especially during the excitement of a relay or contest.

Ring around the Rosie

Skills needed: The dog will follow the participant on lead and "down" on command.

Equipment: None.

Directions: Dogs and participants will walk around the circle reciting the nursery rhyme, "ring around the Rosie, a pocket full of posies, ashes, ashes, we all fall down". At the end of the verse, the participant gives the dog the voice/hand command for "down". The last team down is out of the game.

Variation: 1) Both participant and dog "down."
2) Both participant and dog "sit."
3) Only the participant sits.

Benefits: Attention to task, Directional/positional, Sequencing, Communicating with others, Verbalizing wants and needs, Balance, Mobility, Motor planning, Cooperation/teamwork, Play skills.

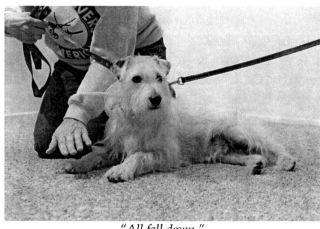

"All fall down."

One-on-One Basketball

Skills needed:	Dog will fetch and drop ball in ring.
Equipment:	2 balls and 2 baskets with adjustable height.
Directions:	"Coach" rolls 2 balls in opposite directions. Participant and dog each go after opposite balls, turn around and go to the basket. 2 points for making the basket on the first try, 1 point for scoring on the second try.
Variations:	1) Game can be played with a "team" of participants competing against a "team" of dogs in a relay fashion. 2) "Team" of participants against one dog. 3) Demo: two dogs compete against each other. You place a tray of balls in the center between the two baskets. The dogs compete against each other to see who can put the most balls in his basket during the allotted time.
Benefits:	Attention to task, Numerical concepts, Sequencing, Balance, Hand/eye coordination, Mobility, Motor planning, Upper body movement/control, Cooperation/teamwork, Play skills.

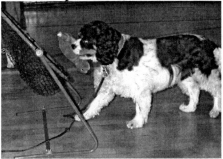

Photo by Linda Grundeman

Riggs slam dunks his toy.

57

Tic-Tac-Toe

Skills needed:	Fetch and drop on command.
Equipment:	Game square divided into nine equal squares spread on the floor. Ten bean bags or toys, five of each color, shape or design ("X" or "O").
Directions:	The game square should be laid on the floor 3 to 6 feet from the "starting line". The participant and the dog alternate throwing/dropping their bean bags on the game mat. First the participant throws his bean bag on the mat and then drops the bean bag for the dog, which the handler directs the dog to fetch and then drop on the mat. The first player with 3 bean bags in a straight line, horizontal, diagonal, or vertical, wins.
Variations:	1) Put the game board in front, right, or left of the participant to work both arms. 2) Require throws to the opposite side of the game board with left hand or vice versa.
Benefits:	Attention to task, Balance, Hand/eye coordination, Motor planning, Range of motion, Upper body movement/control, Cooperation/teamwork, Play skills.

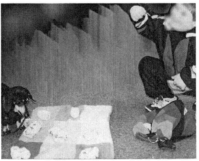

Doozer and friend Playing" Tic Tac Toe."

Dress the Dog

Skills needed:	Dog willing to be handled and tolerant of wearing clothes.
Equipment:	Various hats, shirts, scarves, sunglasses, gloves, socks, etc.
Directions:	Participant chooses articles of clothing to "dress" the dog and puts it on him. Participant must plan/sequence the order of each item of clothing.
Variations:	1) Participants can have a parade or show of their costumed dog. 2) Participants can make up a story about their dog's costume. 3) Can be run as a contest to see who can dress their dog with the most items from a bag of clothing in a specific amount of time. No one is allowed to open their "bags" until the coach/handler says "go."
Benefits:	Attention to task, Sequencing, Caring for others, Safety, Fine motor skills, Hand/eye coordination, Play skills.

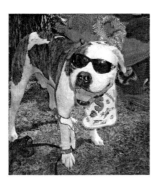 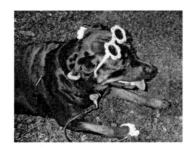 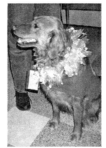

Wrigley, Dutchie and Maui all dressed!

Musical Hoops, Dots

Skills needed:	Walk on lead at slow pace. Will sit on target when music/handler stops.
Equipment:	One hoop/dot per participant placed in middle of the room in a circle.
Directions:	1) Participants will walk around the outside of the circle to the music.
	2) When the music stops, teams will find a target and tell dogs to sit on it. Remove one target.
	3) When music resumes, all teams will walk around the circle again. When music stops, each team finds a target and tells dog to sit on it.
	4) The team left with a target to sit on is eliminated each time, and another target is removed, until only the winning team remains.
Benefits:	Directional/Positional, Verbalizing wants and needs, Balance, Mobility, Cooperation/teamwork, Play skills.
Notes:	No running is allowed.

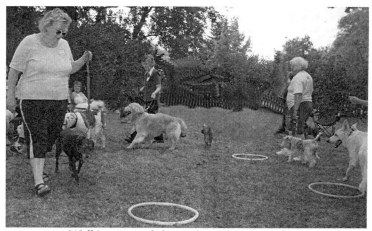

Walking around the circle as the music plays.
(Phoebe, Wrigley, Tyler, Beaner, Apache and Tiberus)

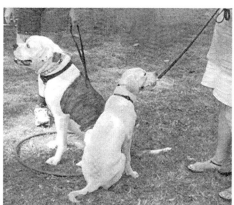
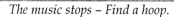
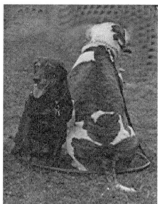

The music stops – Find a hoop.   *It's a Tie!*

What do I Do?

Skills needed: Sit, down, stay, come, and/or additional skills.

Equipment: Hoops or cones to mark a course and any equipment for selected tricks, cards with words or pictures of selected tricks. Cards should be at least 2" x 6" heavy card stock with large print or diagrams laminated to protect against wear and tear.

Directions: The course is labeled with word or picture cards. Participant heels the dog at each cone or hoop, stops and reads the card. Participant gives the dog the command to perform each trick as pictured.

Benefits: Attention to task, Reading, Sequencing, Following verbal instructions, Verbalizing wants and needs, Mobility, Control.

Note: This activity can be modified to work on memory/sequencing as familiarity with the course is achieved.

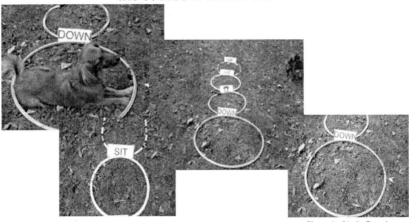

Photos by Linda Grundeman

Beaner plays "What do I do?"

Follow the Leader

Skills needed:	Heel, sit, down, etc.
Equipment:	None-more in the variation of the game.
Directions:	1) Teams walk around the room single file.
	2) Every 30 seconds the instructor calls "stop" and the first team goes to the back of the line and next team is the leader — until each team has a chance to lead the line.
	3) Instructor can have the line stop and participants tell dogs to sit, down, etc.
Variation:	Have first team lead the line through a variety of obstacles — going in, on, under, around a variety of equipment. Equipment can be cones, hoops, dots, chairs, boxes, etc.
Benefits:	Attention to task, Directional/positional, Sequencing, Communicating with others, Following verbal directions, Balance, Mobility, Motor planning, Cooperation/teamwork, Play skills, Self control.

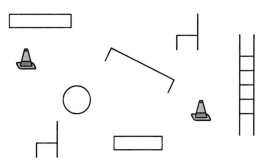

Obstacles may be arranged in any number of ways.

Red Light/Green Light

Skills needed:	Walk on lead, Stop on command.
Equipment:	3" to 4" Red and green cardboard circles. Or, cardboard stop light board with circle cut out.
Directions:	Teams line up on one side of the room, side by side (participant-dog-handler, participant-dog-handler, etc.) The leader stands on the opposite side of the room from the participants with his back to the group and calls "Green light". Once the leader says green light, teams walk towards the leader. Leader quickly turns and says "Red Light" and/or flashes the red cardboard sign. Participants must freeze in place. Anyone caught moving must go back to the starting line. The first team to cross the line wins.
Variations:	The leader faces the competitors' line. On command, "Ready" the game begins and teams follow the direction of the stop light or circles. If the green circle is showing, teams walk towards the leader. If the red circle is showing, teams must freeze (not move at all) and dogs sit. If yellow circle is showing, teams must stop.

Any teams that move on the red light must go back to the starting line. The leader keeps changing the colored traffic lights in random order until one of the teams' participants tags the leader and becomes the winner.

The winner can become the leader of the next game.

Benefits:
Attention to task, Directional/positional, Safety, Following verbal directions, Balance, Mobility, Motor planning, Cooperation/teamwork, Play skills, Self control.

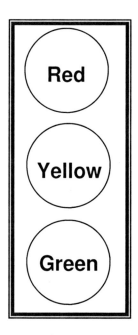

Doggie, Doggie, Where's Your Bone?

Skills needed:	Sit, stay with blindfold and walk calmly at handler's left side while sniffing.
Equipment:	Small puppy milk bones (or any small treat), blindfold for the dog.
Directions:	Participants seated in a circle on chairs, with hands on knees, or seated on floor. Participants pass the treat to their left, while reciting the rhyme (or any other version of this popular rhyme): "Doggie Doggie, Where's your bone? Somebody stole it from your home. Guess who! Maybe you… Maybe the monkeys from the zoo. Wake up doggie, find your bone." The participant holding the treat at the end of the rhyme keeps it, and all participants make a fist and place hands on knees. The dog is then led calmly around the circle at the handlers left side and allowed to sniff each hand. When he finds the bone the participant opens the fist and allows the dog to take the treat from the hand.
Variations:	Dog waits behind door, desk so he can't see. Dog sits in center of the circle with the blindfold on. Participant chooses which dog gets a turn to find the "bone."

Benefits: Communicating with others, Verbalizing wants and needs, Fine motor skills, Hand/eye coordination, Motor planning, Upper body movement/control, Cooperation/teamwork, Play skills, Self control.

Special Comments: This game is one of the very few activities where a circle formation is used. In all other activities it is recommended that participants be seated in chairs or on mats in a semi-circle or a line. When seated on the floor it is best if they sit behind the line, not on it, giving them a visual cue of where to remain. Circles have a tendency to get smaller and smaller and trap you and your dog, getting touched and petted by all from many directions.

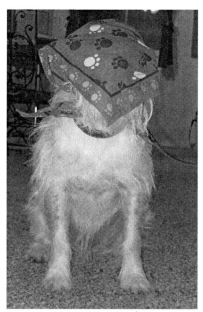

No peeking, Rufus!

Kickball (Doggie Baseball)

Skills needed:	Walk calmly on lead to each base and sit on base when stopped.
Equipment:	Four targets to serve as bases and large soft rubber ball.
Directions:	1) Participants are divided into two teams.

Team one: Participant/handler/dog bat first.

Team two: Participant/handler/dog go to field.

2) Pitcher rolls ball toward home plate

3) Batter kicks the ball, takes the leash and starts walking toward 1st base and then further if possible. Stops at a base to be safe and has dog sit on base.

4) Batter is out if fielder catches the ball on a fly or tags the runner when not on a base.

5) Next batter is up to kick the ball

Scoring: 1 point for every team that touches home after touching 1st, 2nd, 3rd.

Team one bats until they have 3 outs and then team two comes to bat

Benefits: Attention to task, Directional/positional, Numerical concepts, Sequencing, Communicating with others, Balance, Mobility, Motor planning, Range of motion, Upper body movement/control, Cooperation/teamwork, Play skills.

Notes: Only walking on bases and in the field is allowed. Balls that are soft and have minimal roll work best.

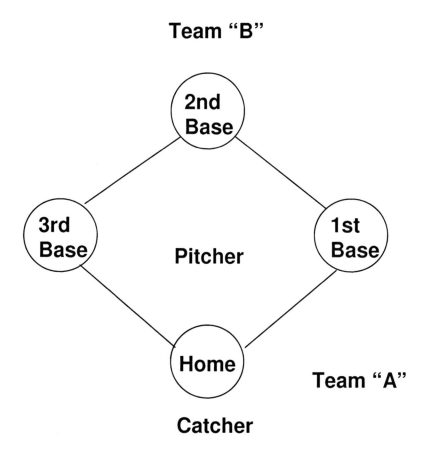

Bowling

Skills:	Fetch ball, find treat, drop ball or knock pins over with nose.
Equipment:	6 bowling pins or styrofoam cylinders. Plastic tray with circles drawn to spot pins. Ball, ring or other object to roll or throw at pins.
Directions:	Participant will roll or throw ball at pins to knock them down. Dog returns ball to participant for 2nd toss. 2nd participant sets up pins. 2nd participant then drops treat in the middle of the pins. 1st participant gives dog command/signal to "Go Bowl." 1st and 2nd participant then switch positions.
Variations:	Score card can be kept if counting and adding are learning goals. Pins and trays can be numbered or lettered if recognition is a goal.
Benefits:	Attention to task, Directional/positional, numerical concepts, Verbalizing wants and needs, Fine motor skills, Hand/eye coordination, Range of motion, Cooperation/teamwork, Play skills.

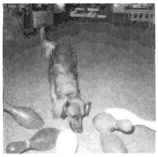

Photo by Linda Grundeman
Bowling with Beaner.

Cup Game

Skills Needed:	To be able to knock over a cup to find the dog treat. "Find it" command.
Equipment:	Set of plastic cups (4 different colors).
Directions:	Participant is given the cups and a treat to hide. Handler prevents dog from looking with blindfold, or goes behind a barrier. After participant sets all the cups up-side down and hides the treat under one cup, the participant tells the dog to "find it."
Benefits:	Attention to task, Color identification, Directional/positional, Sequencing, Verbalizing wants/needs, Hand/eye coordination, Motor planning, Upper body movement/control, Control, Play skills.

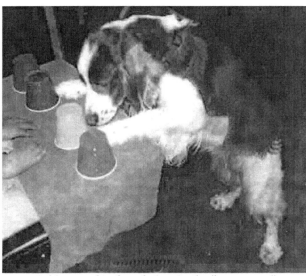

Ashley ponders her choices in the "cup game."

71

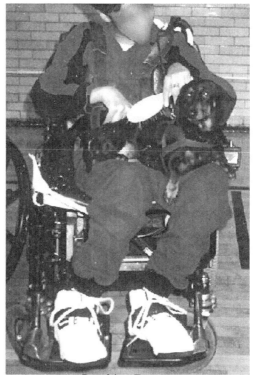

Brushing Doozer.

12

Mastering Daily Living Skills: Motivating with AAT

Special needs individuals have often suffered many years of frustration in the attempt to complete everyday tasks that most of us take for granted. They sometimes try again and again only to fail or to have those around them become impatient and perform the task or skill for them, depriving them the satisfaction and dignity of caring for themselves.

Often, when the same tasks are undertaken in a fun session with an animal assisted therapy team, the excitement of working with a canine friend can create stimulation for the participant and he forgets the difficulties he has previously experienced in completing a particular task. In helping the dog to complete the task, the pressure is off the child himself, and the environment is one of fun where the completion of the task becomes a game for the child to assist his canine partner.

By simulating daily living skills like feeding, getting dressed and cleaning up with the partner and making close approximations of the daily task, the participant will continue to practice over and over with the dog. With each success comes increased self-confidence and determination to succeed. These achievements can literally "jump start" the learning process. The individual no longer associates the completion of these tasks with past frustrations, but now associates them with the games successfully played with his canine partner. With the mastery of some of the basic tasks with the dog, the transference of these new skills to everyday life becomes much easier.

Go to Sleep (Hide the Dog)

Skills needed:	Down, stay.
Equipment:	Small blanket.
Directions:	Participant tells dog to "down" and then "stay". Participant shakes out the folded blanket. Participant covers up the dog for a nap.
Variations:	1) Use blanket and pillow. 2) Have participant completely cover up the dog for a game of "where's the dog." Peek under the blanket and "there's the dog!"
Benefits:	Sequencing, Caring for others, Communicating with others, Verbalizing wants and needs, Motor planning, Upper body movement/control, Play skills.

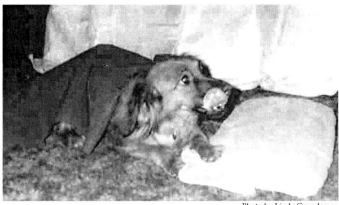

Photo by Linda Grundeman

Beaner prepares for a nap.

Sneeze

Skills needed:	Sneeze on command. Take Kleenex or handkerchief and give to participant
Equipment:	Tissues, wastebasket or bag
Directions:	Give dog command to sneeze. Ask dog if he needs a tissue and offer or point to the box of tissue. Dog fetches tissue for participant to dab his nose. Dog takes the tissue from the participant and drops it in the wastebasket.
Variation:	Participant places box of tissue near dog or places handkerchief in pocket, leaving most of it dangling. Participant pretends to sneeze. Dog gets either tissue or handkerchief, and gives to participant.
Benefits:	Attention to task, Sequencing, Caring for others, Communicating with others, verbalizing wants and needs, Hand/eye coordination, Cooperation/teamwork.
Notes:	If dog sneezes frequently, just add command and praise. Cup hands over dog's nose until he sneezes, add command and praise. Blow on the dog's nose to encourage sneeze, add command and praise.

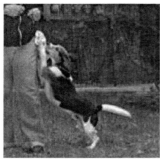
Pretzel grabs the handkerchief.

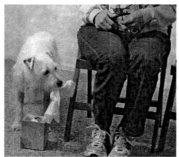
Rufus offers a tissue.

Washing Day

Skills needed:	Fetch, go to.
Equipment:	Rope tied between two chairs, table or wheelchairs, a container of clothespins, a basket of "wash" (socks, gloves or other small items).
Directions:	Participant stands at clothesline. Dog fetches the "wash" from the basket and brings it to the participant. Participant uses clothespins to "hang the wash" on the line.
Variations:	This activity can be run as a relay with the participant leading the dog to the basket to "fetch" the wash and then to the clothesline for the participant to hang before returning the leash to the next participant in line
Benefits:	Attention to task, Sequencing, Verbalizing wants and needs, Following verbal directions, Fine motor skills, Hand/eye coordination, Motor planning.

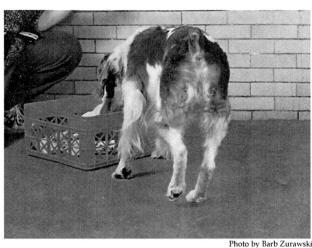

Photo by Barb Zurawski
Ashley helps with the laundry.

Dressing

Skills needed:	Paws up, go to, fetch and drop.
Equipment:	Floppy hat, large gloves or mittens, vest.
Directions:	Participant puts on the gloves loosely with the fingers dangling. (Dog will pull glove off by the fingers so be sure the participant's fingers are clear) Handler sends the dog to the participant with "go to" command. Handler or participant gives dog the "fetch" or "glove" command. Handler gives the dog the command to "drop" the glove in a bag. Dog returns for second glove on command. Clothing is passed to next participant in line while finishing with first participant.
Variations:	1) Add hats and vest for dog to remove. 2) Dog can take items to next participant in line.
Benefits:	Caring for others, Verbalizing wants and needs, Hand/eye coordination

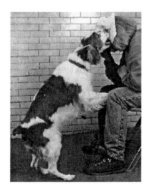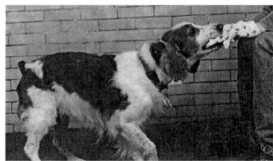

Photos by Barb Zurawski

Ashley helps teach dressing skills

77

Baby Sitting

Skills needed:	Fetch, drop, pull.
Equipment:	Baby buggy, stuffed toy, cloth for blanket, rope (one foot longer than the dog) with a ball or soft toy at the end for dog to fetch. Note that for a small dog, a shoe box can be modified to use as the buggy.
Directions:	Participant throws the stuffed toy "baby" for the dog to fetch and then return to drop in the buggy. Participant gives praise and a treat. Participant throws the "blanket" for the dog to fetch and return to cover the baby. Participant again praises and gives the dog a treat. Participant drops the ball/tug toy attached to the pull rope for the dog to fetch and then walks beside the dog and tells him to take the baby for a walk, ending with praise and a treat.
Variations:	1) Large dogs can fetch the buggy handle to "take the baby for a walk". Handle can be covered in foam pipe insulation available at any hardware store. 2) Dogs who can walk on their hind legs can put front paws on the handle of the buggy and push the carriage.
Benefits:	Sequencing, Caring for others, Verbalizing wants and needs, Hand/eye coordination, Mobility, Motor planning, Upper body movement/control, Play skills.

Ashley Baby Sits

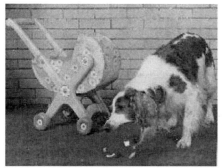
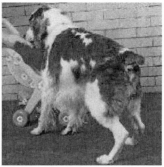

Pick up the "baby."   *Put the "baby" in the stroller.*

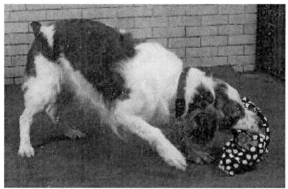

Pick up the "blanket."

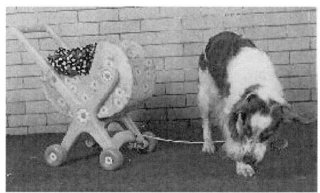

Photos by Barb Zurawski

Take the "baby" for a walk.

79

Treat in the Jar

Skills needed:	Paw.
Equipment:	Plastic jar with screw top lid, fabric pocket with a treat inside.
Directions:	Participant opens the jar and puts a treat in the fabric pocket. Participant replaces the pocket in the jar and *loosely* places the lid back on the jar. Participant places the jar on the floor and holds it while giving the dog the command to open the jar. (Handler should be the one to hold the jar to prevent any possibility of scratching).
Variation:	Handler might store treats in a plastic jar requiring the participant to open the jar each time he rewards the dog, replacing the lid each time.
Benefits:	Attention to task, Sequencing, Feeding skills, Verbalizing wants and needs, Fine motor skills, Hand/eye coordination, Motor planning.
Tip:	You can put a rubber band around the lid to give the dog a bit more traction in unscrewing the lid. You can also use another rubber band to attach the jar to a board for stability and to raise it off the floor for the dog to open.

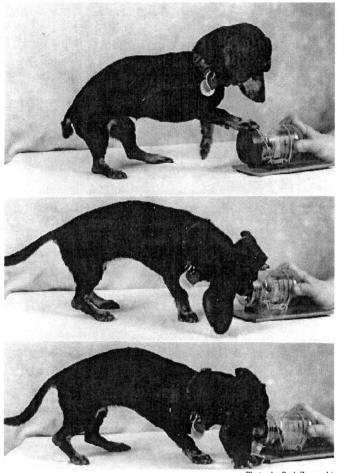

Photos by Barb Zurawski

Doozer opens the jar to get her treat.

Eating Off a Spoon (also a "no trick" trick)

Skills needed:	Sit, stay, gentle treat taking.
Equipment:	Jar, bowl or container for food, small fork or spoon.
Directions:	Participant...

    Tells dog to sit.
    Opens container and places lid on flat surface.
    Picks up spoon.
    Uses utensil to scoop up a single piece of the treat from the container.
    Holds utensil for the dog to gently take the treat.
    Puts down the utensil and replaces the lid on the container.

Variations:	This skill can be made into an entire exercise in meal planning, decision making and cleanup by adding a dish for the dog to be served from and a pan of soap and water for cleanup.
Benefits:	Sequencing, Caring for others, Feeding skills, Safety, Fine motor skills, Control.

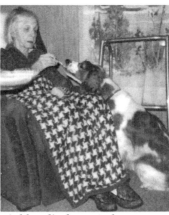

Ashley displays good manners.

Knife/Fork

Skills needed:	Sit, stay, take treat gently from utensil.
Equipment:	Knife, fork, plate, firm bread, hot dog, etc.
Directions:	Give dog command to "sit" next to the table. Give the participant the knife, fork and the plate containing the food to be cut. Assist the participant as needed in the use of the utensils to cut the food in bite-sized pieces for the dog. After the food is cut, the participant should then brush any crumbs onto the plate and dispose in garbage can.
Benefits:	Attention to task, Sequencing, Caring for others, Clean up skills, Feeding skills, Safety, Communicating wants and needs, Hand/eye coordination, Upper body movement/control, Self control
Variation:	Have the participant make sandwiches using firm bread (rye or stale) and a spread (such as squeeze cheese or apple sauce). Select ingredients requiring minimal cleanup and that are in keeping with your dog's dietary needs.

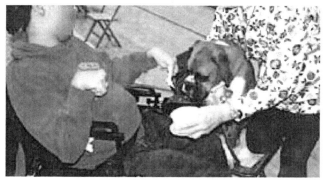

Tootsie carefully takes carrots off a fork.

83

Super "Doo"

Skills needed:	Sit, stand, down and directional commands for positioning. Works best if dog has medium to heavy coat. (Short haired dogs are still great for brushing, hair ribbons, etc.)
Equipment:	Hairclips, bows, foam curlers, dog brush/comb. Any variation of equipment can be used as long as it is safe and gentle to the participant and dog alike. Small dogs can be placed on a table with a non-slip mat or surface.
Directions:	Place dog in comfortable position for the participant to access him. Assist participants in the use of the assorted equipment. These tasks may be performed with a small group or one by one with all steps of grooming being repeated.
Variations:	1) Use a mirror to help with "self" grooming skills. 2) Use a spray bottle for styling, requiring coordination, fine motor skills and sequencing.
Benefits:	Attention to task, Caring for others, Fine motor skills, Motor planning, Play skills,

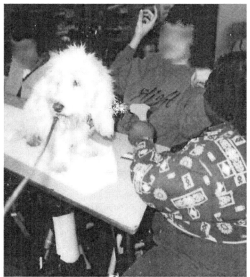

PG gets a new hair "doo."

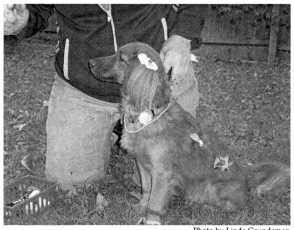

Photo by Linda Grundeman

Beaner patiently waits for his next "bauble."

85

Hide/Find/Cleanup

Skills needed:	Dog must find his toy buried in a box of styrofoam packing.
Equipment:	Toy, box filled with anti-static packing peanuts, broom, dustpan. You will also want to be sure that you have a lid for the box to keep the packing from spilling during transport. Remember, you will have to clean this stuff up, so be careful in your choice of packing material.
Directions:	Participant hides the toy in the packing material. Participant gives dog "find it" command. Dog finds toy in the box and returns it to the participant. Participant uses broom and dust pan to clean up any packing material that spills out of box.
Tips:	1) When starting to teach your dog this trick, place the toy at the top of the packing material. 2) A large shallow bucket can be used for larger dogs.
Benefits:	Sequencing, Clean up skills, Verbalizing wants and needs, Hand/eye coordination, Motor planning,

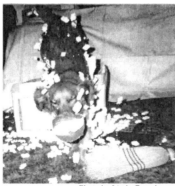

Photo by Linda Grundeman
Beaner finds his toy, then participants practice cleaning skills.

Vacuum Cleaner

Equipment: Broom, styrofoam, wads of paper, wastebasket

Directions: Scatter the wads of paper in a small area. Ask participants to "sweep" the paper towards the basket for the dog to pick up and drop in the basket, being sure to carefully monitor the "swing" of the broom to avoid injury to the participants or the dog. Participant rewards the dog with praise and treat.

Variations: Make a relay of the task where the participant must walk to the "trash," sweep it to the dog for the dog to put in basket. Participant passes the broom to the next participant in line.

Benefits: Attention to task, Sequencing, Clean up skills, Safety, Verbalizing wants and needs, Balance, Motor planning, Range of motion, Upper body movement/control, Cooperation/teamwork, Self control.

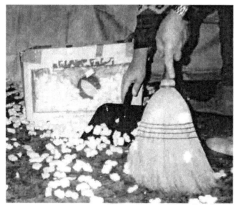

Photo by Linda Grundeman

Cleaning Up.

87

Feed the Dog

Skills needed:	Sit and wait.
Equipment:	Dog bowl, spoon, kibble and second ingredient (such as cottage cheese or yogurt). Be sure all ingredients are safe for your dog's diet.
Directions:	Participant must prepare dog's meal by following the instructions of the handler, opening the containers and measuring out appropriate amounts. Participant mixes the ingredients with the spoon. Participant gives the dog the command to "sit" and then "wait" as he/she places the food on the floor. After the dog finishes his meal, the participant collects the bowls for washing and drying.
Variations:	Mixing several different ingredients extends the activity. Try using measuring spoons/cups to learn quantities.
Benefits:	Sequencing, Clean up skills, Feeding skills, Following verbal directions, Verbalizing wants and needs, Fine motor skills.

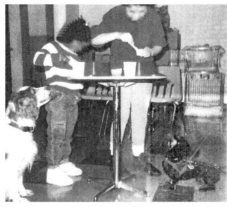

Ashley and Doozer wait for their breakfast.

Take the Dog for a Ride

Skills needed:	Sit, stay, ride in wheelchair, buggy, wagon, etc.
Equipment:	Doll buggy, stroller, wagon, wheelchair, etc.
Directions:	For safety of the dog, the handler places him in the buggy or wheelchair. Participant takes the handle and pushes/pulls it around the room.
Variation:	Costumes can be added.
Benefits:	Attention to task, Caring for others, Balance, Mobility, Motor planning, Upper body movement/control, Play skills, Control

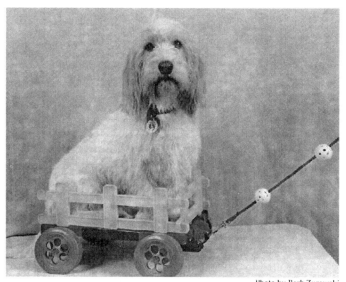

Photo by Barb Zurawski

PG enjoys going for "a ride."

Brush Teeth

Skills needed: Dog must allow others to brush his/her teeth.

Equipment: Extra soft toothbrush, sponge brush and pet toothpaste or breath freshener.

Directions: Participant tells dog to "sit". Participant applies small amount of toothpaste to the brush. Handler holds the dog's mouth and assists the participant with brushing the teeth

Benefits: Attention to task, Sequencing, Caring for others, Verbalizing wants and needs, Fine motor skills, Hand/eye coordination, Control.

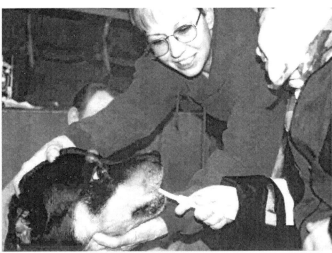

Hildi gets her teeth brushed.

Thinking Ahead—Going Beyond. Other Concepts That Can Be Taught With AAT

With a little creativity and planning, you can use many of your animal assisted activities to teach or awaken a participant's memory to demonstrate various concepts. Colors, numbers, letters, and shapes can easily be combined with various fetching, relay and obstacle activities. For example, "fetch" games can incorporate the naming of a variety of colored balls. The activities on an obstacle course could be numbered. Letters, numbers and shapes can be incorporated in a relay game or in sequencing.

Also, the use of sign language can be re-enforced by having all the dog's tricks cued by both visual and verbal commands. The dog's response to the participant's attempt to sign demonstrates a quick cause and response result and re-inforces the concept of signing.

Most of the individuals you will visit need to increase their communication skills. To that end, it is important to encourage any and all attempts to communicate. Don't demand perfection, but encourage one or two attempts to improve on the original attempt (<u>no more</u>). This applies to all forms of communication whether it is speech, sign, gesture, or picture. The object is to promote and extend the individual's interaction and communication skills.

<u>Sample concepts</u>

top/bottom	some/none	light/heavy
separated/together	in/out	wide/narrow
more/less	her	skip
whole/half	beside	forward/backward
front/behind	match	on/off
and	many/few	corner
most/least	first/last	same/different
row	right/left	first/second/third
big/little	thick/thin	several
full/empty	straight/crooked	moving/still
every	large/small	long/short
beginning/end	flat/thin	rough/smooth
alike/not alike	nearest/farthest	between
dirty/clean	soft/hard	inside/outside
hot/cold	zero	through/around
as many	tall/short	almost
below/above	toward/away	in order
next	loud/quiet	high/low
open/close	slow/fast	away/next to
equal	center	always/never
over/under	up/down	side
middle	flat	before/after

Red/Yellow/Blue

Skills needed:	Take treat gently from participant.
Equipment:	Lolli-pups or colored containers if treats without coloring are preferred.
Directions:	This is a good final or closing activity so that the participant can thank the dogs with praise and treats. Participant asks the handler for the color treat he/she wants to give the dog with verbal/sign or indication of color card. Participant selects the correct color treat and feeds the dog by "making a dish" with his/her hand.
Benefits:	Color identification, Reading, Sequencing, Caring for others, Feeding skills, Verbalizing wants and needs, Fine motor skills.

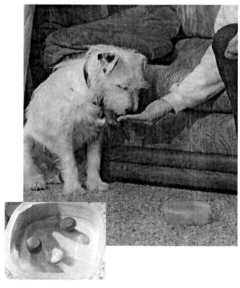

A participant chooses a color for Rufus.

Over/Under, In/On

Skills needed:	Dog must walk with participant on lead and follow participant's commands.
Equipment:	Low 8" jump, hoop, table, bench, cardboard box, etc.
Directions:	Place obstacles around the room or in a line or circle. Participant walks the dog to the obstacle and gives the appropriate command ("over" jump, "under" table, "on" bench, "in" box).
Variations:	1) Can be performed as a relay. 2) Can change positions.
Benefits:	Attention to task, Directional/positional, Sequencing, Verbalizing wants and needs, Balance, Mobility, Motor planning, Control, Cooperation/teamwork.

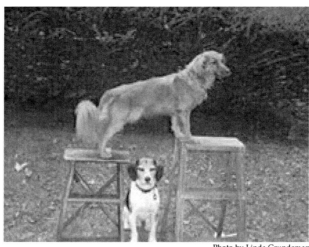

Photo by Linda Grundeman

Pretzel is under; Beaner is over and on.

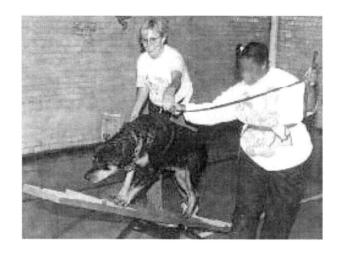

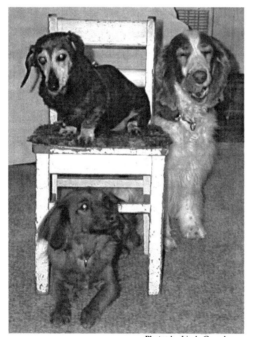

Photos by Linda Grundeman

Hildi, Beaner, Doozer and Keyfer teach positional concepts.

Follow the Dots

Skills needed:	Walk on lead with participant.
Equipment:	Lines, footprints, floor squares with letters, shapes, and colors.
Directions:	Participant will follow the verbal instructions for the course laid out. While walking the course the participant will command the dog to "heel" and "sit."
Variations:	1) Course can be marked with letters or numbers.
	2) Path can be straight, curved or in circles.
	3) Obstacles can be added to the course.
	4) Street signs can be used: stop (octagon), turn (diamond with curved arrow), walk (rectangle), don't walk (rectangle).
Benefits:	Attention to task, color identification, Reading, Sequencing, Following verbal instructions, Verbalizing wants and needs, Mobility, Control, Cooperation/teamwork.

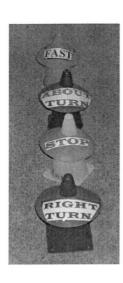
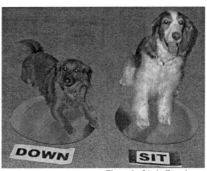

Photos by Linda Grundeman
Beaner and Ashley follow the dots.

Hat Trick

Skills needed:	Sit, down, come, stay, etc.
Equipment:	Hat or bucket, cards printed with simple commands or pictures of a behavior.
Directions:	Participant "heels" dog to hat and draws a card. Participant reads the card. Participant and dog perform the skill on the card. Participant returns the dog to the next participant in line.
Variations:	1) Can be run as a relay. 2) Can begin by pulling one card at a time, and then more cards to promote sequencing activities.
Benefits:	Attention to task, Reading, Sequencing, Communicating with others, Verbalizing wants/needs, Mobility, Control.

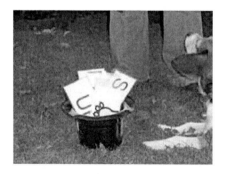

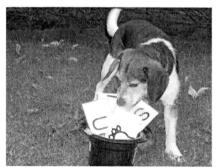

Photos by Linda Grundeman
Pretzel and the Hat Trick.

97

Spelling Bee

Skills needed: Dog must know the tricks that will be spelled.

Equipment: None, or handler/participant's choice.

Directions: Participant calls dog's name and spells the command (i.e., S-I-T, D-O-W-N, C-O-M-E).

Variations: 1) Foreign language
2) Signal only

Benefits: Reading, Communicating with others, Verbalizing wants and needs, Control.

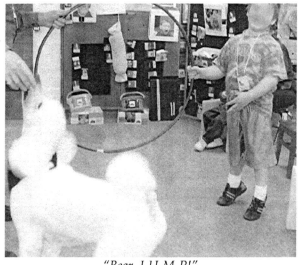

"Bear, J-U-M-P!"

Mail Person

Skills needed:	Take/fetch and target, drop and/or fetch/give and go to.
Equipment:	Letters and mailbox.
Directions:	Participant gives the dog a letter and commands the dog to go to the mailbox. At the mailbox, the participant gives the command to drop the letter.
Variation:	Dog can take the letter out of the box and deliver it to the participant.
Comment:	This is a good game to use for the holidays (Christmas, Valentine's Day)
Benefits:	Attention to task, Sequencing., Communicating with others, Verbalizing wants and needs, Control.

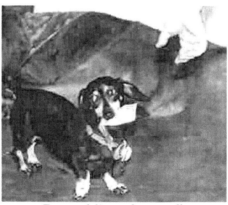

Doozer delivers the payroll.

Where's the Dog?

Skills needed:	Sit, down, stay.
Equipment:	Based on position selected.
Directions:	Place dog in "sit/down, stay" in a positional relationship to something/someone in the room. Participant must communicate (sign, utter, say, picture) where the dog is. When correct, participant gives the dog a treat.
Variations:	1) Positions are unlimited (examples include on, in, under, next to, in front) 2) Words can be made up with pictures. For example, the (picture of dog) is (picture of dog "sitting") in the (picture of chair). 3) Have the participant place the dog and then explain where the dog is. 4) Use a variety of places for the same position. 5) Use a variety of positions for the same phrase
Comment:	It is important to build the participant's confidence and accept any attempt at communication of the command by the participant. Reinforce the participant's attempt by reiterating where the dog is (i.e. "Oh! The dog is IN the hoop") and adding the sign or picture.
Benefits:	Attention to task, Directional/positional, Communicating with others.

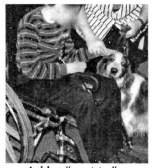

Ashley "next to."

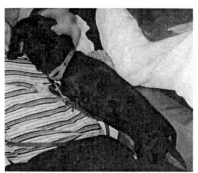

Doozer "on."

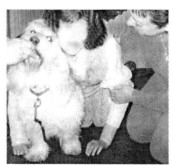

PG "under."

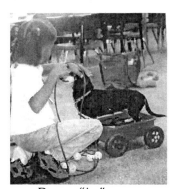

Doozer "in."

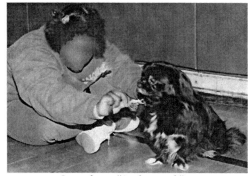

Sassafrass "in front of."

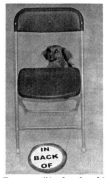

Beaner "in back of."

Roll the Tire

Skills needed:	Dog must walk with the participant and follow commands.
Equipment:	Small tire (bicycle or motorcycle)
Directions:	While participant is rolling/holding the tire, the participant tells/signs the dog to go through the tire, turn and come back through the tire (in, out, in, out, etc.)
Variations:	1) A hula hoop can be used in place of the tire. 2) Change the words to "go, come" or "left, right." 3) Can be run as a relay.
Benefits:	Attention to task, Directional/positional, Sequencing, Verbalizing wants and needs, Balance, Motor planning, Upper body movement/control.

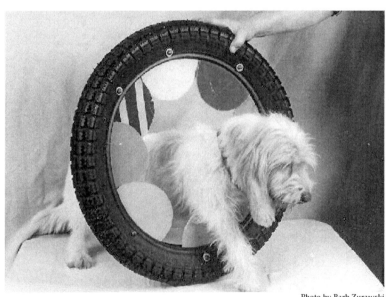

Photo by Barb Zurawski

PG demonstrates "through the tire"

Read those Labels

Skills needed:	Scent discrimination.
Equipment:	6-12 different grocery items, colored blocks, or empty pop cans taped closed.
Directions:	Spread items in an area. Ask the participant to name their favorite item from the tray. Ask the dog to retrieve the item. Allow the dog to walk around the participant with the chosen item.
Comment:	This is basically a "trick" used for demonstrations, but can be used effectively during visits.
Benefits:	Color identification, Verbalizing wants/needs, Control.

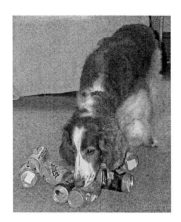 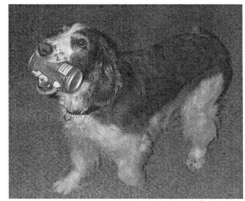

Photos by Linda Grundeman

Keyfer "reads the labels" to select the correct flavor.

Meditate

Skills needed:	Paws up, sit/stay.
Equipment:	Chair.
Directions:	Tap chair and give the "paws up" command, the "stay" command, and then "meditate" (where the dog lays his chin on the chair or puts his head down between his paws). Give "done" command and dog gets off the chair.
Comment:	This is basically a "trick" used for demonstrations, but can be used effectively during visits.
Benefits:	Attention to task, Sequencing, Verbalizing wants/needs, Control.

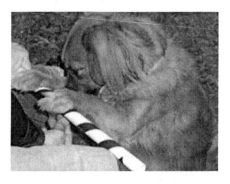

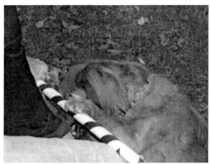

Photos By Linda Grundeman

Beaner "meditates."

14

Only the Beginning

I truly hope that this book will become a stepping off point to stimulate your ideas. You can work with participants to motivate them in areas they are working on such as: physical movements, language, cognition, self help, attention and visual skills. Through activities they also develop responsibility and confidence.

I hope that this will help to motivate teams to look beyond the basic activities of petting, brushing, fetching, and walking. Your own new and creative activities will help participants to reach greater heights and will encourage even more individuals to reach for new horizons with AAT.

Remember to learn from the participants, other teams, and your dog. Search for those additional and creative ways that you can better impact the lives of everyone you come in contact with. Always be open to challenging yourself and maximizing your sessions.

Remember that this all started with an idea over 20 years ago with the purpose of bringing happiness, comfort, diversion, self confidence and skill mastery to individuals facing a variety of challenges.

Look what we've started.

Now where can you take it?

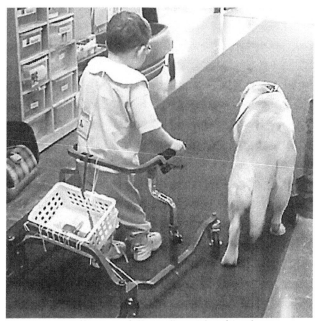

Mellow carefully walks with a friend.

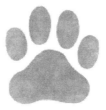

Acknowledgments

There is no way to thank the oh so many individuals who brought this book to fruition. I'd like to let all know that they are sincerely appreciated and without them this book would have not made it to completion.

Many thanks to all my two-footed and four-footed friends who provided the encouragement, stimulus and motivation to put these ideas on paper. These include:

- The dogs who taught me.

- The children who inspired me and showed me the way. They encouraged me to develop activities through their interest and creativity and at times, taught the dogs new tricks.

- The friends who gave me the courage to think that I could do this and the support and encouragement to complete this book.

The opportunity to be able to participate in an activity which makes a difference in another's life has been a life-changing experience for which I will be forever grateful. I have been surrounded by the kindness of so many teams. Their willingness to step forward and make that extra effort provides opportunities for the many individuals we visit. These teams give participants new experiences and opportunities to try skills which they had long given up trying to master. Not a session goes by without the people we work with prodding us to search for new and better ways to do animal assisted therapy activities.

These teams have my gratitude for giving me the opportunity to share countless activities with program participants over the last twenty-two years. It is those individuals who have been my motivation, inspiration, and innovative spark to search for and create new activities that benefit so many with special needs.

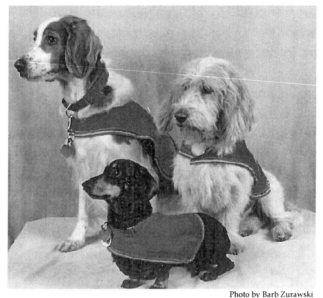

Photo by Barb Zurawski

Ashley, PG and Doozer
My original "three musketeers"
who courageously pioneered my future.

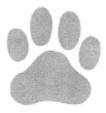

Appendix

The following charts should be considered a guideline for the activities/games that I have found to be effective for promoting a particular benefit or skill.

For instance, if a participant's goal is to improve self care or feeding, use the Daily Living Charts to locate those skills and activities that can be used to promote mastery in those areas. Page numbers for the activities are cross-referenced on each chart for your convenience.

By using your own skills and creativity you will most certainly generate even more benefits from any given activity.

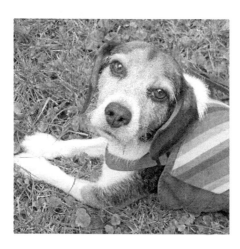

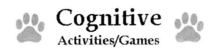

Cognitive
Activities/Games

Page	Activity/Game	Attention to Task	Color Identi- fication	Directional/ Positional	Numerical Concepts	Reading	Sequencing
25	Give Kiss						
26	Nothing Trick			X			X
28	Play Piano	X		X			X
29	Play Tambourine	X		X	X		X
30	Motorcycle Rider			X			
31	Read	X				X	X
37	Ladder Walk	X		X			
38	Hoop	X		X			
39	Pulling Wagon	X		X			
40	Weave (Izzy Dizzy)	X		X			
42	Catch	X		X			X
43	Snake Walk	X		X			X
44	Carry the Basket	X		X			
45	Over/Under	X		X			X
46	Jump Rope	X		X	X		X
47	Crawl	X		X			X
48	Slide	X		X			X
49	Dance						
50	Dice				X	X	X
56	Ring Around the Rosie	X		X			X
57	One on one Basketball	X			X		X
58	Tic Tac Toe	X					
59	Dress the Dog	X					X
60	Musical Hoops			X			
62	What do I do?	X				X	X
63	Follow the Leader	X		X			X
64	Red light-Green Light	X		X			
66	Doggie, Doggie						

110

Activities to Motivate and Inspire

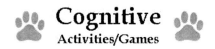

Cognitive
Activities/Games

Page	Activity/Game	Attention to Task	Color Identi-fication	Directional/ Positional	Numerical Concepts	Reading	Sequencing
68	Kickball	X		X	X		X
70	Bowling	X		X	X		
71	Cup Game	X	X	X			X
74	Go to Sleep						X
75	Sneeze	X					X
76	Washing Day	X					X
77	Dressing	X					
78	Baby Sitting						X
80	Treat in Jar	X					X
82	Eating off Spoon/fork	X					X
83	Knife/Fork	X					X
84	Super "Doo"	X					
86	Hide/Find/Clean-up						X
87	Vacuum Cleaner	X					X
88	Feed the Dog						X
89	Take the dog for a ride	X					
90	Brush Teeth	X					X
93	Red/Yellow/Blue		X			X	X
94	Over/Under, In/On	X		X			X
96	Follow the Dots	X	X			X	X
97	Hat Trick	X				X	X
98	Spelling Bee					X	
99	Mail Person	X					X
100	Where's the Dog?	X		X			
102	Roll the Tire	X		X			X
103	Read those Labels		X				
104	Meditate	X					X

111

Daily Living
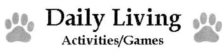
Activities/Games

Page	Activity/Game	Caring for Others	Clean up Skills	Feeding Skills	Safety
25	Give Kiss				
26	Nothing Trick				
28	Play Piano				
29	Play Tambourine				
30	Motorcycle Rider	X			
31	Read				
37	Ladder Walk				
38	Hoop				
39	Pulling Wagon				
40	Weave (Izzy Dizzy)				X
42	Catch				
43	Snake Walk				
44	Carry the Basket				
45	Over/Under				
46	Jump Rope				
47	Crawl				
48	Slide				
49	Dance				
50	Dice				
56	Ring Around the Rosie				
57	One on one Basketball				
58	Tic Tac Toe				
59	Dress the Dog	X			X
60	Musical Hoops				
62	What do I do?				
63	Follow the Leader				
64	Red light-Green Light				X
66	Doggie, Doggie				

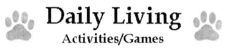
Daily Living
Activities/Games

Page	Activity/Game	Caring for Others	Clean up Skills	Feeding Skills	Safety
68	Kickball				
70	Bowling				
71	Cup Game				
74	Go to Sleep	X			
75	Sneeze	X			
76	Washing Day				
77	Dressing	X			
78	Baby Sitting	X			
80	Treat in Jar			X	
82	Eating off Spoon/fork	X		X	X
83	Knife/Fork	X	X	X	X
84	Super "Doo"	X			
86	Hide/Find/Clean-up		X		
87	Vacuum Cleaner		X		X
88	Feed the Dog		X	X	X
89	Take the dog for a ride	X			
90	Brush Teeth	X			
93	Red/Yellow/Blue	X		X	
94	Over/Under, In/On				
96	Follow the Dots				
97	Hat Trick				
98	Spelling Bee				
99	Mail Person				
100	Where's the Dog?				
102	Roll the Tire				
103	Read those Labels				
104	Meditate				

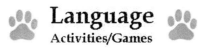

Language
Activities/Games

Page	Activity/Game	Communicating with others	Following verbal Directions	Verbalizing wants and needs
25	Give Kiss	X		X
26	Nothing Trick			X
28	Play Piano		X	X
29	Play Tambourine	X	X	X
30	Motorcycle Rider			X
31	Read	X		
37	Ladder Walk			X
38	Hoop	X		X
39	Pulling Wagon	X		X
40	Weave (Izzy Dizzy)	X		X
42	Catch	X		X
43	Snake Walk	X	X	X
44	Carry the Basket	X		
45	Over/Under	X	X	
46	Jump Rope	X		X
47	Crawl	X	X	X
48	Slide	X		X
49	Dance			X
50	Dice	X		X
56	Ring Around the Rosie	X		X
57	One on one Basketball			
58	Tic Tac Toe			
59	Dress the Dog			
60	Musical Hoops			X
62	What do I do?		X	X
63	Follow the Leader	X	X	
64	Red light-Green Light		X	
66	Doggie, Doggie	X		X

Language
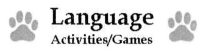
Activities/Games

Page	Activity/Game	Communicating with others	Following verbal Directions	Verbalizing wants and needs
68	Kickball	X		
70	Bowling			X
71	Cup Game			X
74	Go to Sleep	X		X
75	Sneeze	X		X
76	Washing Day		X	X
77	Dressing			X
78	Baby Sitting			X
80	Treat in Jar			X
82	Eating off Spoon/fork			
83	Knife/Fork			X
84	Super "Doo"			
86	Hide/Find/Clean-up			X
87	Vacuum Cleaner			X
88	Feed the Dog		X	X
89	Take the dog for a ride			
90	Brush Teeth			X
93	Red/Yellow/Blue			X
94	Over/Under, In/On			X
96	Follow the Dots		X	X
97	Hat Trick	X		X
98	Spelling Bee	X		X
99	Mail Person	X		X
100	Where's the Dog?	X		
102	Roll the Tire			X
103	Read those Labels			X
104	Meditate			X

Motor
Activities/Games

Page	Activity/Game	Balance	Fine Motor Skills	Hand/ Eye Coordi-nation	Mobility	Motor Planning	Range of Motion	Upper Body Movement/ Control
25	Give Kiss							
26	Nothing Trick							X
28	Play Piano					X		X
29	Play Tambourine		X	X		X		X
30	Motorcycle Rider	X			X	X		X
31	Read		X					X
37	Ladder Walk	X			X	X		X
38	Hoop					X	X	X
39	Pulling Wagon	X			X	X		X
40	Weave (Izzy Dizzy)	X			X	X	X	X
42	Catch			X	X	X	X	X
43	Snake Walk	X			X	X		
44	Carry the Basket		X	X				
45	Over/Under	X			X	X	X	
46	Jump Rope							X
47	Crawl	X			X			
48	Slide				X	X		X
49	Dance	X		X			X	X
50	Dice							X
56	Ring Around the Rosie	X				X	X	
57	One on one Basketball	X		X	X	X		X
58	Tic Tac Toe	X		X		X	X	X
59	Dress the Dog		X	X				
60	Musical Hoops	X			X			
62	What do I do?				X			
63	Follow the Leader	X			X	X		
64	Red light-Green Light	X			X	X		
66	Doggie, Doggie		X	X		X		X

Motor
Activities/Games

Page	Activity/Game	Balance	Fine Motor Skills	Hand/ Eye Coordination	Mobility	Motor Planning	Range of Motion	Upper Body Movement/ Control
68	Kickball	X			X	X	X	X
70	Bowling		X	X			X	
71	Cup Game			X		X		X
74	Go to Sleep	X				X		X
75	Sneeze			X				
76	Washing Day		X	X		X		
77	Dressing			X				
78	Baby Sitting			X	X	X		X
80	Treat in Jar		X	X		X		
82	Eating off Spoon/fork		X					
83	Knife/Fork			X				X
84	Super "Doo"		X	X		X		
86	Hide/Find/Clean-up			X		X		
87	Vacuum Cleaner	X				X	X	X
88	Feed the Dog		X					
89	Take the dog for a ride	X			X	X		X
90	Brush Teeth		X	X				
93	Red/Yellow/Blue		X					
94	Over/Under, In/On				X	X		
96	Follow the Dots				X			
97	Hat Trick				X			
98	Spelling Bee					X		
99	Mail Person					X		
100	Where's the Dog?							
102	Roll the Tire	X				X		X
103	Read those Labels							
104	Meditate							

Social

 Social

Activities/Games

Page	Activity/Game	Control	Cooperation/ Teamwork	Play Skills	Self Control
25	Give Kiss				X
26	Nothing Trick	X			
28	Play Piano	X		X	
29	Play Tambourine	X	X	X	
30	Motorcycle Rider	X		X	
31	Read	X	X		
37	Ladder Walk	X	X		
38	Hoop	X			
39	Pulling Wagon	X	X	X	
40	Weave (Izzy Dizzy)	X	X	X	X
42	Catch	X	X		
43	Snake Walk	X			
44	Carry the Basket		X		X
45	Over/Under		X		X
46	Jump Rope	X	X		
47	Crawl	X	X		
48	Slide	X	X		
49	Dance	X			
50	Dice	X	X	X	
56	Ring Around the Rosie		X	X	
57	One on one Basketball		X	X	
58	Tic Tac Toe		X	X	
59	Dress the Dog			X	
60	Musical Hoops		X	X	
62	What do I do?	X			
63	Follow the Leader		X	X	X
64	Red light-Green Light		X	X	X
66	Doggie, Doggie		X	X	X

Social
Activities/Games

Page	Activity/Game	Control	Cooperation/ Teamwork	Play Skills	Self Control
68	Kickball		X	X	
70	Bowling		X	X	
71	Cup Game	X		X	
74	Go to Sleep			X	
75	Sneeze		X		
76	Washing Day				
77	Dressing				
78	Baby Sitting			X	
80	Treat in Jar				
82	Eating off Spoon/fork	X			
83	Knife/Fork				X
84	Super "Doo"			X	
86	Hide/Find/Clean-up				
87	Vacuum Cleaner		X		X
88	Feed the Dog				
89	Take the dog for a ride	X		X	
90	Brush Teeth	X			
93	Red/Yellow/Blue				
94	Over/Under, In/On	X	X		
96	Follow the Dots	X	X		
97	Hat Trick	X			
98	Spelling Bee	X			
99	Mail Person	X		X	
100	Where's the Dog?				
102	Roll the Tire				X
103	Read those Labels	X			
104	Meditate	X			

About the Author

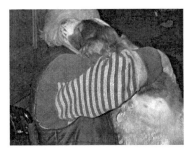

With a BA in Special Education and Physical Education, Nancy Lind spent 27 years as a special needs teacher. During that time she was introduced to animal assisted therapy, and was so taken with the concept that she pioneered a program for her own students. Creating activities with the dogs for her students, she was astounded at the skills they were able to master with the help of a canine friend...skills that were seemingly out of reach prior to the introduction of the dogs. The results were overwhelming, and the program was so well received that it led to the addition of several "teams" visiting on a regular basis.

With a desire to share what she learned from her students, Nancy founded Rainbow Animal Assisted Therapy (a not for profit 501c3) in 1987. Today, Nancy is the CEO of Rainbow Animal Assisted Therapy, which has grown to over 200 teams involved in over 100 programs, among them schools, hospitals, libraries, rehabilitation centers, etc. She is still actively involved in all aspects of the organization, particularly member education.

She is a Certified Delta Animal Evaluator, as well as a Registered Delta Pet partner. In addition, she is a certified tester for Therapy Dogs International, Inc., and a temperament tester with the American Temperament Society.

She continues to create and implement activities that motivate and inspire for more effective animal assisted therapy in a variety of settings.

LaVergne, TN USA
10 December 2009
166572LV00004B/4/P